The Rules of
"NORMAL"
EATING

A Commonsense Approach
for Dieters,
Overeaters, Undereaters,
Emotional Eaters,
and Everyone in Between!

Karen R. Koenig, LICSW, M.Ed.

The Rules of "Normal" Eating:
A Commonsense Approach for Dieters,
Overeaters, Undereaters, Emotional Eaters,
And Everyone in Between!
©2005 by Karen R. Koenig

Gürze Books
P.O. Box 2238
Carlsbad, CA 92018
(760) 434-7533
www.gurze.com

Cover design by Abacus Graphics, Carlsbad, CA

Library of Congress
Cataloging-in-Publication Data
Koenig, Karen R., 1947-
    The rules of "normal" eating: a commonsense approach for dieters,
    overeaters, undereaters, emotional eaters, and everyone in between!
/ Karen R. Koenig.-- 1st ed.
        p. cm.
    ISBN 0-936077-21-2 (alk. paper)
    1. Eating disorders--Prevention. 2. Obesity--Prevention. 3. Food--
Psychological aspects. 4. Food habits--Psychological aspects.
    I. Title.
    RC552.E18K64 2005   2004027862
    616.85'2605--dc22   CIP

NOTE

The author and publisher of this book intend for this publication to provide accurate information. It is sold with the understanding that it is meant to complement, not substitute for, professional medical and/or psychological services.

6 8 0 9 7

This book is dedicated to my father,
who made me believe I could.

CONTENTS

ACKNOWLEDGMENTS

My feeling of gratitude to the many people who encouraged me to become a writer and who helped me write this book is surpassed only by my joy in having the opportunity to publicly thank them. Thanks to all my students and clients for trusting me to help them with their food problems, deepening my understanding of our complicated and conflicted relationship with food and each other, and proving over and over that we do not have to remain victims of our hungers.

Appreciation goes to my three original manuscript readers, Nina Case Martin, Beth Mayer, and Emily Fox-Kales, who gave me the feedback I needed to take my rough draft forward, as well as to Audrey Ades, Alice Rosen, Rivka Simmons, and Marilyn Unger-Riepe of the Greater Boston Collaborative for Body Image and Eating Disorders for their invaluable support throughout the writing process.

I have been fortunate to work with Janice M. Pieroni, consultant/entertainment attorney, who has been nothing but encouraging about my writing, enthusiastic about this book, and patient with my literary anxieties. *The Rules of "Normal" Eating* is equally fortunate to have found a nurturing home at Gürze Books with Lindsey Hall Cohn and Leigh Cohn, whose dedication and contributions to the field of eating disorders deserve praise of the highest order.

To Lynda Pasqua: special thanks for being there throughout all my struggles, eating and otherwise, and for always having the knack of making me feel better. To Keith Loring, my husband: your quiet belief in me made this book possible.

INTRODUCTION

B ack in the days when I was either starving or stuffing myself, who would have dreamed that I'd find myself counseling, teaching, and writing about how disordered eaters can become comfortable around food by learning a set of rules for "normal" eating. By the way, the quotes around "normal" underscore that there's no one particular way to eat, but rather, a range of appropriate eating behaviors that reflect our weight, appetite, metabolism, biochemistry, lifestyle, and activity level. The quotes are to remind you to find comfortable eating habits based on who *you* are. Copying someone else's "normal" eating is like cheating on a test: the results may look good, but you don't learn a thing and only end up fooling yourself.

Although I was never the type of chronic dieter who jumped on every diet bandwagon, for more than 20 frustrating years I alternated between rigidly restricting my food intake and succumbing to food frenzies that broke my heart and my spirit. Gaining and losing the same 10 to 20 pounds over and over, I hated myself when I was overweight and lived in fear of my fat self when I was slim. Sound familiar?

Then in the early 1980s I picked up the book *Fat Is a Feminist Issue*, by Susie Orbach, and my eating changed forever. The book became my bible, my map, my compass, my lantern in the dark, my crutch, my guru, the finger prodding me from behind and beckoning me forward. It introduced me to a revolutionary way to relate to food—by actually listening to and trusting my body—and I spent the next decade learning and diligently practicing the behaviors and attitudes that "normal" eaters take for granted.

I began the amazing process of learning to trust my body to guide my eating by reading every book I could find on making peace with food and finding a natural weight. I also entered therapy, which deepened, broadened, and accelerated the process of discovering what I needed to change about myself to become a "normal" eater. A few years later, I was hired by a Massachusetts-based, cutting-edge psychoeducational venture called the FACE program (Focus Awareness on Chronic overEating). As a facilitator for them, I continued to learn about and fine tune my own eating.

During the next 10 years, I earned my master's degree in social work and began teaching adult education classes for compulsive and restrictive eaters, counseling students who wanted additional help, and writing articles on overcoming disordered eating. Currently I have a private psychotherapy practice, teach eating awareness classes to the public, and lead seminars for my colleagues in local graduate continuing education programs on how to treat clients with compulsive, emotional, and restrictive eating problems.

I think of myself as a "normal" eater about 90–95 percent of the time. Because of my dysfunctional relationship with food for three-plus decades, I accept that I might never eat like someone

Second, diets and extended restriction of food fly in the face of your metabolic needs because they're based on external, arbitrary, punishing rules that deny and betray your body's natural mechanisms for feeding and nourishing itself. Third, such artificial constraints evoke an overwhelming sense of physical and emotional deprivation that only increases the distrust you already feel toward your body.

Contrary to public opinion (and maybe your own opinion as well), there is no such thing as failing at dieting because you can't be a failure at something that was unreasonable and impossible to achieve to begin with. I am barely five feet tall. If someone tried to shame me for being unable to touch the ceiling, I'd think they were crazy because that expectation is so obviously ridiculous. The same is true of dieting and caloric restriction as a permanent approach to eating. The *real* failure is the assumption that anyone would willingly deny themselves the joys and pleasures of food as a way of life. You might as well lock yourself in jail and swallow the key!

Worse than being downright ludicrous, the idea of ongoing, extreme restriction of food is emotionally dangerous and physically debilitating. Adhering to a strict diet plan for more than a few weeks is nearly impossible (as well as being a total drag as soon as the initial high of white-knuckle control wears off), and you end up blaming yourself as soon as you take your first no-no nibble. Each diet failure erodes a little more trust and confidence in your ability to feed yourself. Lacking faith, you wind up turning to yet another diet as your salvation, a cycle that is truly vicious.

The other end of the spectrum, living as a fugitive from dieting, is equally painful. Lacking internal constraints around food, you may believe that there's something gravely wrong with you.

Obsessed with thoughts of what you should and shouldn't eat, you drown yourself in guilt, shame, disgust, self-contempt, and all-consuming self-loathing. When you look around and see other people eating "normally," you blame yourself for your inability to feel relaxed and comfortable around food, for not having the discipline you believe you should have. If you gain weight from excessive eating, use laxatives, or purge, your self-esteem plummets even lower and your shame doubles. You've added one more reason to hate yourself. No matter how well things are going in any other part of your life, you never feel quite normal or successful, and that becomes your secret shame and sorrow.

Whichever end of the eating spectrum you're on—chronically overeating or undereating—you are suffering unnecessary pain and misery. This book will help you relieve some of it. It won't solve all your problems, but it will improve your self-esteem, give you a sense of power over your life, teach you to honor your emotional and physical needs, help you trust yourself, and free up your emotional energy for more productive and enjoyable living.

This book is for you if you:

- don't think you're a "normal" eater and want to find out how to become one
- are thin or fat or yo-yo wildly between weights
- eat emotionally (to avoid feeling) or compulsively (without awareness)
- are afraid of food and feel guilty and ashamed when you eat what your body craves
- have been chubby since childhood
- put on unwanted pounds after your first child or your last period

- won't allow yourself to say yes to food or can't figure out how to say no
- are tired of dieting, bingeing, or checking the scale each day to see what you can and cannot eat
- want to live at a comfortable body weight without feeling deprived of food's pleasures
- love and want to help someone who is obsessed with eating or not eating
- believe you can have a healthier relationship with food

This book teaches an approach to behavioral transformation that has a proven, well-documented track record in the treatment of conditions such as depression, anxiety, and substance abuse. Cognitive-Behavioral Therapy focuses on three aspects of your relationship with food that you'll need to change to become a "normal" eater: 1) what you believe, 2) what you feel, and 3) how you behave. Because all three are essential and interrelated, you must work attentively on each area to reach your eating goals. It's not enough to modify your habits, which are only external manifestations of your thoughts and feelings. For lasting change, you will have to dig deeper and reexamine and revise what Alcoholics Anonymous so aptly calls your "stinkin' thinkin'." After all, you wouldn't plant a garden on a toxic waste dump.

A few words about what this book is not. It's not a quick fix for eating problems. If you're looking for a magical pill to cure your food problems, I hope you kept the receipt for this book. It took years to develop your dysfunctional relationship with food, and it will take some time (realistically, many months to a few years) to establish healthy beliefs and behaviors.

This book is also not a guide to nutrition. Although feeding your body the right nutrients is absolutely essential to good mental and physical health, focusing on nutrition at this point, before you are well on your way to becoming a "normal" eater, would only confuse you and short-circuit the recovery process. After you've become a more "normal" eater, you will have plenty of time to focus on nutrition. That means waiting until your new beliefs and behaviors have taken hold and you're in touch with your body's hunger, craving, enjoyment, satisfaction, and fullness signals and have become comfortable and adept at choosing foods that satisfy you. If you're concerned about not getting adequate nutrients from food, visit a registered dietician to find out what vitamins, minerals, and supplements you should be taking. Then take them religiously.

The concepts and changes I propose in the pages ahead are simple but not easy. Becoming a "normal" eater may well be one of the hardest things you do in your life. I can't predict how long the process will take or how many setbacks you'll have along the way, although I know that your progress will come in fits and starts and that you'll relapse and make mistakes until you've learned all you need to know. The one thing I guarantee without hesitation is that on your journey toward "normal" eating, every new healthy belief, every authentic feeling, and every changed behavior will give you a better life and a safer, saner relationship with food.

Karen R. Koenig, LICSW, M.Ed.

1

THE RULES OF "NORMAL" EATING

Oh, Good, Rules!

A client with a compulsive eating problem told me early in her therapy about an incident that had astonished her so greatly that she was still in awe a week later. At the dessert bar of a free buffet, a colleague she didn't know very well turned to her and said, "I just don't feel like having anything." My client, on the other hand, had been trying to figure out how many desserts she could haul back to the table without dropping anything. She simply couldn't fathom how this woman, who looked like she could easily afford the calories, could turn down dessert, especially when it wouldn't cost her a penny. I explained that her colleague might not have been hungry or in the mood for something sweet, that she might be a "normal" eater.

Shaking her head in amazement, my client gasped, "A normal eater? What's *that*?"

What is a "normal" eater?

If you've been a compulsive, emotional, or restrictive eater for any length of time, you know that you don't eat "normally." As a *compulsive eater*, you eat mindlessly, without thinking about your actions, groping your way through a bag of chips while watching TV, grazing through the cabinets in your kitchen without even realizing it, polishing off a box of Raisinettes in the car on the way home from work. As an *emotional eater*, you automatically reach for food in response to uncomfortable feelings. After a fight with your partner, you suddenly return to earth when your spoon hits the bottom of the ice cream container, or you gather all your favorite foods around you for comfort to make Saturday night a little less lonely. Most, but not all, people who eat too much are both compulsive and emotional eaters.

As a *restrictive eater*, on the other hand, you probably know more about calories and fat grams than many registered dieticians do. You keep yourself on a permanent, lifelong diet leash and rarely let go. Filled with shame and guilt around food, you're terrified of gaining weight and follow rigid rules about when and how much you can eat. You use your relationship with food to manage your problems and feelings.

Many disordered eaters career wildly between overeating and undereating—within a day (barely eating all day, they gorge at night) or a week (severely restricting food on weekdays and bingeing on weekends), or by punctuating weeks or months of strict dieting with weeks or months of chaotic compulsive/emotional eating.

If any of these patterns fit you, you know that you feel anything but "normal" around food. To you, "normal" eaters are alien creatures filled with magical powers who think food is nothing but, well, food. Who are these amazing human-looking beings who are in tune with their bodies and make bizarre comments like, "I'm not hungry right now," "No, thanks, I'm done," and "Jeez, is it lunchtime already?" How can they be so unafraid of food, think so lovingly of it, and nonchalantly comment, "Boy, am I hungry. I can't wait to dig in," "I can't remember the last time I tasted something so delicious," and "I'd love a little more, thanks."

What are "normal" eaters? Do they eat only at salad bars and shop at health food stores, shunning white flour and simple carbohydrates? Do they sit at a table to eat three square meals a day and never snack? Do they never overeat or undereat? Is everyone who's neither overweight nor underweight a "normal" eater? And most important, how do they do it?

The fact is, there is no one right way to be a "normal" eater. "Normal" eaters share similar attitudes toward food, but some eat two big meals a day because of large appetites and tight schedules, while others nosh every few hours and feel pleasantly satisfied all day long. Some are picky fussbudgets around food and make sure the waiter gets their order exactly right, while others eat practically anything. Some are nutrition-conscious label scanners, while others couldn't tell a carbohydrate from a catamaran. Some don't mind skipping a meal if they're busy, while others pay exquisite attention to satisfying their food cravings and believe nothing beats a good meal. Some rarely overeat because food simply doesn't mean that much to them, while others expect to overeat on special occasions and think nothing of it. (No, getting out of bed each morning does *not* constitute a special occasion!)

How much, how little, or how often a person eats does not define whether or not they're a "normal" eater. What "normal eaters" have in common is that they don't think in terms of *good* and *bad* foods, as if slabs, scoopfuls, wedges, chunks, slices, nuggets, and morsels from the kitchen are little angels or devils with agendas of their own. "Normal" eaters are aware that there are high- and low-calorie foods and may even occasionally consider caloric content in choosing what to eat. Many enjoy being healthy and eating nutritiously. However, they don't base their choices solely on how many calories or fat grams a particular food has. Most "normal" eaters really enjoy food and eating. And it would never occur to them to weigh their food—or constantly think about weighing their bodies!

"Normal" eaters respond to a set of conscious and unconscious rules relating to food. Yes, *rules*. Many people think that only diets have rules. In fact, what terrifies compulsive and restrictive eaters alike is the thought that without dieting, there would *be* no rules and caloric chaos would reign! Not true. In fact, far from it.

What are the rules of "normal" eating?

The rules of "normal" eating are deceptively simple. Excepting unusual circumstances, "normal" eaters:

1. Eat when they are hungry or have a craving
2. Choose foods they believe will satisfy them
3. Stay connected to their bodies and eat with awareness and enjoyment
4. Stop eating when they are full or satisfied

In short, they tune in to their body's signals that they need food for fuel or have a yen for a particular something. They respond to and respect their hunger, then choose foods based on what their body says it wants or doesn't want. They don't try to satisfy themselves with somebody else's idea of what will ring their chimes. They don't expect food to be orgasmic, but they do aim for enjoyment by staying connected to their taste buds and their feelings of fullness and satisfaction. When they've had enough (we'll get to what *that* means later on), they stop eating. Eating in this way is as natural to them as breathing. The key point here is that for "normal" eaters, saying yes or no to food is no big deal.

How do I know if I'm hungry?

When I speak of hunger, I mean the general sense that there's a lack of fuel in the system and you're running on empty. Signals of hunger include a gnawing or hollow sensation in the chest cavity or stomach area, light-headedness, growling in your belly, slight irritability, perhaps a mild headache, and even a vague physical queasiness that's difficult to describe. Hunger is a biological phenomenon, and its sensations grow gradually stronger. Hunger is not just wanting to chew or swallow or fill your mouth with food. We'll get to what that is later.

Knowing your hunger level is essential to "normal" eating. If you're so hungry that you're nauseous or ready to eat dirt, you've waited too long and will probably inhale every bit of food in your general vicinity. If you're not at all hungry, you won't know when to stop because you were full or satisfied to begin with. Not surprisingly, food tastes most enjoyable when you are moderately hungry. How clever that we are designed in such a logical way!

Here is what true hunger is not: an ache in your soul. The feeling you get when you don't want to do something. Thirst or exhaustion. Any kind of emotion that drives you to food. Stuffing down uncomfortable feelings. *If it can be satisfied by something other than food, it is not hunger.*

What is a food craving?

Food cravings are callings that need to be answered, itches that need to be scratched. The idea is to stop scratching as soon as the itch goes away; that is, identify the craving and eat exactly as much as you need to satisfy it. Food cravings are different from hunger, and they may or may not accompany it. Both are physical sensations, stirrings from deep inside our bodies. Hunger tells you it's time to eat, and cravings tell you what to eat.

So what exactly is a craving? It's a yen for a particular taste or food that comes on suddenly, seemingly out of the blue—an organic longing for something as general as sweet, sour, spicy, tart, or salty, or as specific as a fresh raspberry or eggs Florentine. With a craving, sometimes you can actually taste the food in your mouth when it isn't there! Your mouth waters for it. Occasionally, I can taste kiwi fruit on my tongue when I am nowhere near one. That's a craving (and also a little weird, I know). I'm not a big meat eater, but every two years or so (probably when I haven't been eating enough protein), I find myself dying for spareribs or a hamburger. The craving can be so fierce that, much as I adore my husband, he'd be putting himself in mortal danger by standing in front of the car when I'm ready to peel out in search of red meat. That's an honest-to-goodness craving.

You will not necessarily have a craving every time you're hungry. Sometimes you'll know exactly what you want at practically the instant you realize you're hungry. Other times, you'll wander around the kitchen or supermarket or stare at the menu while your dinner companions grow impatient before you can make a selection.

Here is what a craving is not: You have nothing to do, so you decide to eat. You want to fill the emotional or spiritual void inside you. You're sad or disappointed and convince yourself that eating will pick up your spirits. You're unsettled by having a sliver of leftover birthday cake in the refrigerator. Cravings are not rooted in emotional discomfort. They are biological, not psychological, independent from your feeling state, and, like hunger, are truly about food.

How do I know what foods will satisfy me?

If you've been dieting or restricting your food intake for ages, you may have temporarily lost the capacity to know what foods your body truly wants. You will have to figure it out by trial and error. The first question is, of course, how hungry you are. If you're very hungry, you may want something heavy and substantial; if you're just getting hungry, you may want something lighter. You may need to sit quietly and let an image of a particular food float into consciousness and settle into your mouth. If you're at a restaurant, look over the menu a few times, pausing at each item to attend to whether or not your body flickers interest. Or look through your kitchen to see what's available, not in a frantic way, but calmly, imagining what each food would taste like. If you have too many choices and feel confused—or if nothing strikes your fancy—try asking the following questions:

- Do I want something sweet, salty, sour, hot, mushy, lumpy, cold, thick, liquidy, creamy, crunchy, soft, hard, chunky, frozen, bitter, icy, bland, bulky or spicy, starchy or sugary, filling or light?

- Do I feel like not chewing and want the food to effortlessly slide down my throat, or are my teeth looking for action?

The way to select food that satisfies is to look for answers inside yourself, not in a diet plan or on a food scale. Whatever you choose will depend on your mood, what's available, the setting you're in, what you've already eaten that day, and what you expect to eat later on. Think of it, you are the only person in the entire universe who knows what you want to eat!

"Normal" eaters don't get bent out of shape if the restaurant is out of their favorite dish. They order something else and hope that the item will be available next time. They try to choose satisfying foods, but if they don't feel satisfied, they don't stuff themselves out of frustration with some dish they didn't want in the first place. *Au contraire*: if the food isn't satisfying, they eat less of it!

Here is how choosing satisfying food does not happen: You make your selection based exclusively on caloric or fat content. You order the least fattening item on the menu. You order the most fattening item on the menu. You eat only salad until you feel yourself sprouting bunny ears and whiskers. You're starving or weren't hungry to begin with. You make a choice based on what you think you should or shouldn't eat. You're very upset or angry. You order whatever the person you are with orders.

No matter how long you've been silencing that voice inside you that knows just what food will hit the spot, it has not forsaken you. You may have to ask it to speak up and coax it out, and you certainly will have to listen very carefully. But if you're persistent, that voice will rise joyously in you, grateful to finally be heard.

What does it mean to be connected to my body and eat with awareness and enjoyment?

If you've ever had great sex, you know what it feels like to be connected to your body. You're full of heavenly sensation, glad to be alive, thrumming, exquisitely awakened by your lover's every touch. You are 100 percent there. Your body is screaming yes, yes, yes! If you've ever had mediocre sex, you know what it feels like to disconnect from your body. That's when you start calculating your car payments, wondering when you're going to find time to pick up your suit from the cleaners, or worrying whether your mother got her prescription filled. You have unconsciously (or maybe consciously) flipped your switch to off. You are barely there.

While your hands and mouth are eating, where are your thoughts? Are you purposely avoiding thinking about the food because you're afraid of it? Are you counting calories or wondering what food will arrive next? Is your body at the table while your mind is back at the office? Staying connected to your body while you're eating means focusing on two things and two things only: the food and your body, your body and the food. If you're eating alone, this may not be so difficult—unless, of course, you're reading, watching TV, talking on the phone, working at the computer, playing with the cat, or distracting yourself from your body-food connection in some other mundane way.

"Normal" eaters automatically (unconsciously) check in with their bodies even when they're eating and doing other activities. They are multitasking without losing touch with how their body is responding to food because their procedural memory is at work. Procedural memory lays down patterns—what we call learning—when we aren't even aware that we're making these unconscious connections. In this case, memory has paired eating with body cues established in infancy and childhood. "Normal" eaters maintain an unconscious connection between food and body even when they appear to be focused on the latest gossip or absorbed in a documentary on the Civil War. They're in tune with their body's signals because the signals are strong and clear, because they've been listening to them for a long time and have learned to trust them, and because they interpret them correctly.

Unconscious behaviors of "normal" eaters when they are eating include:

- They breathe regularly.
- They chew their food well before swallowing it.
- They look up from their plate often.
- They pause and enjoy the taste of what they are eating.
- They put their fork or spoon down occasionally and don't think of utensils as extensions of their arm.
- They have a silent, automatic, back-burner dialogue with themselves regularly while eating to see if they are still hungry or have reached fullness or satisfaction.
- They focus on the food in front of them, not what they ate yesterday or what they will be eating tomorrow.
- They don't care what's on someone else's plate or imagine that anyone cares what's on theirs.

Here is how *not* to stay connected to your body while eating:

- Shovel or gobble your food.
- Guilt trip, shame, or hate yourself for what you are eating or what you ate earlier.
- Eat as much as the person next to you.
- Tell yourself that you don't deserve to eat.
- Eat as little as the person next to you.
- Forget to breathe or taste the food.
- Rush through the meal.
- Struggle not to eat anything.
- Eat when you are too stressed to enjoy food.
- Worry while you're eating.
- Feel self-conscious about what you're eating.
- Eat to please someone else.

Are feeling full and satisfied the same thing?

The sensations of feeling full or satisfied are distinct but interrelated physical reactions to the experience of eating. They are often viewed as identical and are frequently confused. If you haven't eaten in several hours, feel light-headed and queasy, and are embarrassed by the racket in your stomach, you are experiencing hunger; that is, your body needs to fuel up on food. Think of hunger as signaling an absence of food in the body and fullness as its opposite, signaling a presence of sufficient food in the body. Fullness is a *quantitative* measurement.

Satisfaction is a *qualitative* measurement and may have nothing to do with how much you've eaten. You may feel satisfied after a few bites, or you may not feel you've reached satisfaction after a seven-course meal. Satisfaction may or may not accompany fullness.

For example, imagine that you're eating a tuna fish sandwich. Here are some possible responses you might have:

- *Feeling satisfied without feeling full.* Before you reach a state of fullness, you may have had enough of the taste of tuna and feel satisfied. You may still be hungry and not yet full, but no longer want tuna fish.

- *Feeling full without feeling satisfied.* You may no longer feel hungry and may have eaten enough in terms of quantity, but feel unsatisfied because you either didn't enjoy the sandwich or did enjoy it, but now crave another taste.

- *Feeling full and satisfied.* The tuna sandwich filled you up nicely and you're licking your chops in satisfaction, desiring nothing more to eat.

- *Feeling neither full nor satisfied.* Because you were ravenous, the sandwich only made a dent in your hunger and you are not yet full. You didn't particularly care for the taste of tuna, so you're left feeling unsatisfied.

There's another circumstance when you may be seeking only satisfaction, not fullness, from food: when you aren't hungry in the first place, yet you crave a particular food. Let's imagine that you're sitting at your desk working away and have a sudden urge for, say, a sourball. You're hardly looking to fill your belly with sourballs, but there is something inside you that is screaming *tart-citrus-sweet*. When you have a craving, the focus is on taste and texture. If you suck slowly on the sourball, it's more than likely that you'll need only one or two to satisfy your craving, and that will be that.

Here are two simple equations that will help you decide whether you should be seeking fullness or satisfaction.

- Hunger + food = satisfaction and/or fullness
- Craving + the craved food = satisfaction

The general rule of thumb regarding fullness and satisfaction is this: both fullness and satisfaction are healthy responses to hunger, while satisfaction is the only appropriate response to a craving. A craving—if you are authentically connected to your body and savor your food choice—should bring you to an "aahh" place with fairly little food. That doesn't mean that you may not want more of it; if it tastes good, you very well may. It merely means that more is not going to bring you increased flavorful enjoyment. In fact, the opposite is true: if you eat with awareness, you will reach a pinnacle of enjoyment (satisfaction) and after that, the food will not taste as good. And, remember, sometimes you may be *satisfied* but will continue to eat because you're still hungry.

There's no way that you need a pint of ice cream to satisfy a craving; if a few spoonfuls or a dish don't do the trick, then ice cream isn't what you were craving to begin with. Remember, with a craving you're going for a peak experience that should result in a natural diminishment of the original desire. Try to honor your food cravings and not ignore them. Learn to differentiate between mouth hunger, which is generally emotional, and genuine cravings, which are more biological. Becoming a "normal" eater means saying yes to authentic cravings and enjoying eating.

How will I know when I have had enough?

When Donna Summer belts out the lyric "Enough is enough is enough," she's describing a situation that has reached its end point—in this case, a love affair. Actually, the lyrics of the song imply that Ms. Summer has had more than enough, that she's had too much. Unfortunately, it's not always easy to know exactly when enough *is* enough—enough love, creature comforts, stress, money, praise, work, play or leisure, intimacy, space, sleep, drink, emotional or physical pain—or food. We tend to overdo or underdo, then overdo and underdo again, struggling to find that elusive point that says "Just right."

At other times we may not realize that we know what is enough without even thinking about it. On days we can sleep in, we may feel rested or still sleepy when we wake up. If we've had enough sleep and feel refreshed, we get up. If not, we roll over and head back to dreamland. With little or no analysis and reflection, we depend on our body to give us an accurate reading of what to do.

The same is true of other everyday activities. We can't wait to curl up on the couch and lose ourselves in the latest bestseller; yet after a while our body says "Enough" and signals us to finish the chapter and find something else to do. Or we may be on vacation, content to do absolutely nothing. So how come after days or weeks of lounging and mindless activity, we yearn for something more meaningful and start to look forward to returning home? Or, working on a project hour after hour, we finally give up and sigh, "That's all for now." The point is that, if we listen, our body-mind will speak.

Each person's sense of *enough* in relation to any activity is unique. What's enough TV for you may be too much or too little for me. Enough runs on a ski slope or enough sets of tennis will be different for each individual, depending on a number of complex factors. A finely tuned sense of what is enough in life is truly a remarkable and useful gift. It signals that you are in balance, in sync with your body and mind.

When you lose touch with your body's needs and wants, you can't sense when it's had enough of anything, especially food. The problem of not knowing when you've eaten enough to feel full or satisfied stems from childhood. If, as a child, you were allowed and encouraged to tune in and respond to your body's signals for satisfaction and fullness, then you'll grow up to be an adult who trusts the accuracy of your internal messages. If you said you were done with your macaroni and cheese, and your parents took away your half-eaten food with a smile, they were validating and reinforcing your body's cues regarding enough food. Now, after years of practice, you'll be skilled at identifying satiation.

If, on the other hand, someone (Mom? Dad? Grandma? Grandpa?) ignored or challenged your bodily signals of fullness and satisfaction, you'll grow into an adult who cannot recognize such signals or who willfully ignores or overrides them. If someone in your childhood overtly or covertly gave you the message to disregard your body cues and keep eating or stop eating, this may have taught you to depend on external factors to tell you how much to eat. You learned to base your sense of enough on some*thing* outside yourself—portion size, whatever you can get away with, calories or fat content, what you feel you deserve—or some*one* outside yourself—the approval or disapproval of a parent, spouse, friend, partner, co-worker, or whoever is watching you eat.

The more you depend on external cues to tell you anything about your relationship with food, the farther away you move from being a "normal" eater. You can't hear what your body is saying when you're listening hard to someone else's appraisal, whether that voice is real or inside your head. If you enjoy the sound of the waves, you need to move nearer the ocean. If you want to hear, really hear, your body's signals, you have to be more closely connected to them and block out everything else. Only then will you learn when enough is enough.

Moreover, if you have problems determining whether you're satisfied or full, you may also experience similar difficulties with the concept of enough in other areas. With both intimates and strangers alike, you may find yourself alternately giving too much or too little. You may not know when to stop working or how to take adequate time for yourself. You may deprive yourself of essential things while overdoing it on nonessentials. If excess and deficiency, that is, the concept of too much or too little, is a theme in your life, learning what is enough food is an excellent way to begin to return to a healthy equilibrium. Achieving balance in your life, having enough of this and that, depends on saying one of the two simplest words in the English language at just the right times.

How do I know when to say yes and when to say no to food?

Two of the earliest words we learn as children are yes and no. Generally we have learned to say them by the age of two or three. As we grow older, we acquire synonyms and euphemisms for yes and no, but the duo still remains a fundamental, emphatic expression of our thoughts, feelings, needs, fears, and deepest desires. When feminists of the 1970s wanted to communicate to men that women had the right to reject unwanted sexual advances, they came up with a simple message: "*Yes means yes, and no means no*". Short, easy to pronounce, with meanings that are unequivocal, the words yes and no are packed with power. Consider the fact that hearing them may fill us with immense joy or infuse us with intense sadness—or may even go so far as to make us want to live or die.

As a practicing psychotherapist, I often think that much of what mental health practitioners identify as emotional problems or dysfunctional personalities stems from what I call a basic yes-no disorder, which means saying yes and no at the wrong times. Too many people get it exactly backwards: they say yes (and display moving-toward behavior) when they should be saying no, and they say no (and display moving-away behavior) when they should be saying yes. They gravitate toward people who are likely to harm them emotionally and retreat from people who are likely to help and support them. They say yes to self-destructive actions and no to life-supporting ones.

Nowhere is the imbalance and misapplication of yes and no more apparent than in the food arena. In fact, we might say that restrictive and compulsive/emotional eating boils down to a basic problem of saying yes and no at the exact wrong times. Restrictive eaters almost always say no to food, whereas compulsive/emotional eaters almost exclusively say yes. Both are out of balance with their wants and out of touch with their needs. The no sayers are afraid of excess, while the yes sayers fear deprivation. "Normal" eaters say yes and no to food at the appropriate times—appropriate because they trust their body to tell them the truth about what it needs, in a more or less balanced way.

If you are a restrictive eater struggling to get to "normal," your goal is to say yes to food on more occasions. If you are a compulsive/emotional eater, your goal is to say no more often. If you alternate between being a restrictive eater and a compulsive/emotional eater, you're essentially ping-ponging back and forth between periods of too much yes and too much no. Your goal is to seek a reasonable balance.

Thinking in terms of increasing and decreasing yes and no responses to food may seem simplistic or even silly. Becoming a "normal" eater obviously involves more than automatically responding appropriately one way or the other when feeding yourself. However, thinking in terms of more or less yes and no can help point you in the right direction and move you toward feeling more balanced when you're around food. It will also give you practice in pushing yourself through the discomfort of doing more of what is good for you and less of what is bad. As you learn to say yes and no more appropriately to food, it will be easier to respond more appropriately in other areas of your life. Getting yes and no in the correct balance is an integral part of healthy self-care.

2

THE RULES OF CHANGE

Can't It Just Happen While I'm Sleeping?

Now that you've learned the Rules of "Normal" Eating—eating when you're hungry or have a craving, choosing satisfying foods, staying connected to your body and eating with awareness and enjoyment, and stopping eating when you're full or satisfied—your anxiety level may be skyrocketing and you may be filled with despair. So much to change, so little time: how will I ever get eating right? You may be wishing for a magic pill so that you could awaken tomorrow morning a perfectly tuned "normal" eater. You may even be feeling so anxious right now that you're thinking about heading to the kitchen for a little nosh.

Food is not the answer to anything but hunger and craving, and there's no miracle that will transform you into a "normal" eater. There are, however, aspects of behavioral change that are important to understand as you embark on the journey of learning to eat "normally." I call these the Rules of Change. Once you accept the idea that transformation is an incremental process and recognize how change occurs, you'll be clearer and feel more relaxed about the adventure ahead.

What are the Rules of Change?

Sometimes we change inadvertently, unconsciously, whether we want to or not. We're shaped by learning outside our awareness every minute we're alive; our brains are constantly soaking up new information. Anything can act as a change agent, even when we don't realize it. For example, say you decide to trade in your old sedan for an SUV. You may not recognize that your itch for an SUV was stimulated by seeing the roads filled with them and your desire to be like everyone else, or even that you're partial to a particular model because of the way it was pitched on TV.

The Rules of Change do not describe this kind of subliminal change that is outside your awareness. On the contrary, if you're going to attempt the 180° turnabout you'll need to become a "normal" eater, you can't rely on unconscious change. Far from it. Transforming your relationship with food will take nothing less than total awareness of your beliefs, feelings, and behaviors, along with tons of courage and a doggedness you may never before have felt for reaching any goal. This kind of change is like giving birth to a new self, a brand new you, and it is an extremely labor intensive endeavor, both mentally and emotionally.

If you're up for the challenge of your life (followed as surely by reaping the most bountiful rewards you can imagine), here are the Rules of Change:

1. Change is simple but not easy.
2. Change is incremental.
3. Change is slow.
4. Change doesn't happen without discomfort.
5. Change is facilitated by having or developing specific personality traits.
6. If you put one foot in front of the other, you can't help but get to where you want to go.

Why is change only simple, not easy?

Somehow, perhaps through hearing it over and over and because the phrase is catchy, we've learned to string together the words "simple and easy." The pairing is often used in instructions and directions and may be accurate when describing how to put up a tent or throw together a quickie cake mix recipe. In this book, I have tried to present theories and practices for changing eating behaviors in straightforward language and to break them down into manageable steps that don't require a degree in rocket science. In fact, you may read some of my ideas and think, Wow, that's simple!

However, if behavioral change were *easy*, we'd all be happy and healthy—and I'd be out of a job. The reality is that true, lasting transformation is often hard, hard, hard. I probably should have included that last sentence as the first Rule of Change, but I was afraid you might feel so discouraged that you'd give up before you even got started.

What is incremental change?

Think two steps forward, one step back. I'm always amazed when a client comes in with a hangdog expression on her face and tells me that nothing is changing in her life. Change is hard, she complains, and she'll never reach her goals, eating or otherwise. Then in the next breath she offhandedly mentions that she has done something that impresses me as utterly phenomenal and that I know will help her get unstuck and move forward. My job is to help her notice how her speedometer is in reality inching up when she's dying to go from 0 to 100 in no time flat.

Here are some examples of incremental behavioral change: You're thinking of leaving your partner and you start sleeping in another room. You burn all your diet books. You buy a treadmill. You refuse to respond to someone who's yelling at you. You tell the person who cuts in front of you in line in the supermarket that "Yes, you *do* mind." You make a dental appointment. You call a friend when you're upset. You buy a book on how to discipline your unruly child. You join a support group. You cut up your credit cards. You stop thinking about calories and eat because you're hungry. You join an on-line dating service. You sign up for an evening class. You eat two of your favorite cookies instead of the whole bag. You make an appointment with a therapist. I could go on and on, but you get the point. The person who buys a treadmill isn't fit *yet*. The one who makes a dental appointment hasn't achieved *perfect* dental care. The one who brings home a book on unruly children hasn't become a *model* parent. The point is that all these people are taking steps in the direction of their goals by doing something positive.

So many compulsive/emotional and restrictive eaters practice all-or-nothing thinking. Do you? If so, that's one reason you may have fallen so easily into the diet mentality that promises complete success in breakneck time (and convinces you that a plan is "simple and easy" to follow, to boot). If you continue to think of yourself as either a failure or a success, I can almost guarantee that you won't achieve "normal" eating. It took you decades to become a compulsive/emotional or restrictive eater, and it will take time—truthfully, most likely a couple of years— to become truly comfortable with healthy, "normal" eating habits. But each day, with each food interaction, you can make incremental change.

The key is to acknowledge every tiny change and make a big whoop of a deal about it, praising yourself to the skies for each and every minuscule move you make in the right direction. My guess is that this might be a foreign experience for you, that usually you minimize your progress and maximize your mistakes. I have a hunch that you're used to mentally dragging yourself over burning coals every time you binge, eat when you're not hungry, or don't take time to choose satisfying foods. You notice what you're doing wrong more than what you're doing right. Incremental change demands that you ratchet up your atten- tion to take in each and every forward movement.

Why is change so slow?

If I were a neurobiologist, I would answer by giving you com- plicated data on how the brain registers behavior and how, at a cellular level, habits are laid down. Suffice it to say that habits do get patterned in our brains through an intricate system of neural pathways, whether or not we are conscious of learning. What you need to remember in terms of changing your eating is that the more we do something (thinking, feeling, or behaving), the stronger the neural pathway grows. The less frequently we do something, the weaker the pathway. If we stop doing something completely, the neural pathway withers out of existence.

On a subclinical level, our brain doesn't judge what's good or bad for us. It works like a sponge, sopping up what it hears and sees and feels, and squeezing it into our memory bank. Whether we reinforce good learning habits when studying for an exam or reinforce bad ones and sneak off to play computer games, our brain just keeps establishing neural pathways. Think of the brain as a nondiscriminatory, equal opportunity neural pathway builder! So when we put off tasks we don't want to do, lie to ourselves, or engage in negative self-talk, the brain lays down tracks, creating patterns and habits of procrastination, denial, and self-criticism. With every repetition, the thought, feeling, or behavior gets reinforced.

Here's a graphic way to understand change. Picture a hill of damp sand with a marble on top. If you give the marble a nudge in one direction, it will roll down the hill, forming a slight groove in the sand. Each time the marble gets nudged in the same direction, it will slide into the groove and the groove will deepen until you only have to place the marble on top of the hill for it to plop right into the groove and plunge downward.

Now suppose you decide that you want the marble to roll down the *other* side of the sand hill. You'll have to place the marble on top of the hill and push it in the other direction because if you don't, it will slip automatically into its old groove. If you push it only once or twice in the new direction, its inclination will still be to return to its old groove. So initially you'll need to push the marble in the new direction over and over until a new groove is carved out. Eventually when your old groove and the new groove are about even, the marble will have the potential to roll either way. To ensure that it will always go in the new direction, you'll have to keep gently nudging it until the old groove fills up with sand and the new groove is deeply carved. Then the marble will naturally fall into the new groove every time.

Translating this marble analogy into behavioral terms, we have to repeat a new behavior more often than an old behavior in order to have the new one become a habit and the old one disappear. Behaviorists call this process *conditioning* because it conditions or prompts us to behave in certain ways. Of course, most people are not linear learners and don't go straight from point A to point B. We try a new way, revert back to the old way for a while, then tentatively try the new way again. We're inconsistent, then we wonder why we're not changing quickly enough, after all our hard work.

Think back to the marble on the sand hill. What would happen if sometimes you pushed it one way and sometimes you pushed it the other? The old and new grooves would stay about even, right? That's what happens when you try a new behavior or way of thinking, then return to the old action or thought. For example, if food makes you anxious, you try pushing yourself to eat when you're moderately hungry. Succeeding, you feel proud of overcoming your fear. But the next time you feel hunger pangs, you ignore them and put off eating until you are nearly sick. Or you triumphantly pass by the jar of chocolate kisses on your co-worker's desk one day, only to find yourself sneaking a handful the next. Alternating like this for days, weeks, months, or even years causes you to feel as if you'll never change even though you're doing things right a good deal of the time. You prevent yourself from changing by reinforcing both the new *and* the old, achieving a behavioral draw.

Returning to the marble analogy, we could say that every time you revert to an old behavior, you're deepening the first groove, while every time you push yourself to practice a new behavior, you're not only carving the second groove more deeply, but you are allowing sand to erase the first one. Similarly, if you continue to press onward with a new behavior, the neural pathway in your brain that elicited the old behavior will eventually fade away.

There's another reason that change is excruciatingly and annoyingly slow. Psychologically, we like the familiar. We find comfort in thinking of ourselves in a certain way and maintaining a stable identity. If we were to change overnight, it would cause such internal chaos and confusion about ourselves (never mind how startled other people would be), that we'd barely be able to function. Think how you feel when you're thrown into a new situation or role, even one you may be looking forward to, such as a promotion or marriage. Initially, you feel discombobulated and unsure of yourself until you can integrate your new perception of yourself with your old or until, over time, one slowly replaces the other. On a more superficial level, think how strange it is to look in the mirror after you've made a drastic alteration in your appearance—for example, radically changing your hairstyle. Disoriented, you keep looking at yourself, checking for signs of recognition!

Now imagine that the change you're trying to make is regarding one of your most basic relationships, the one you have with food. One day you're a binge eater feeling miserable about yourself because you can't decide if food is your best friend or your worst enemy, and the next day it's easy as pie to eat "normally." One week you're petrified of gaining an ounce and refuse to eat anywhere but at home, and the next week you want to eat out for every meal. Quick change might sound enticing and exciting, but I guarantee that if it happened, your head would be spinning and you'd feel wildly out of control because you wouldn't know who you were. Nor would others. Better that you become a "normal" eater more gradually so that your old self and your new self have time to integrate.

Why do I have to be uncomfortable in order to change?

Here's an exercise you can do that will answer the question. Notice how you're sitting, but don't change your position. Focus on any parts of your body that aren't quite comfortable. Your arm may have fallen asleep, you may have a crick in your neck, or your legs may be crossed in an awkward manner. Once you've located some discomfort, shift slightly to a more comfortable position. That's it, that's the exercise.

What did you learn? I hope you noticed that you needed to be both *uncomfortable* and *aware* of your discomfort in order to change your position. Absorbed in reading this book and directing your full attention to it, you might have been sitting uncomfortably for quite a while without noticing it. That's perfectly normal. You had to become aware of your discomfort for it to disturb you enough to shift positions.

I know from having led this exercise many times in my eating awareness classes that you may have scanned your body and found no points of discomfort. You felt just fine the way you were sitting. This suggests that you had awareness (of your body) but no actual discomfort, so there was no reason for you to change your position. That's OK too.

This exercise demonstrates the equation:

DISCOMFORT + AWARENESS = CHANGE.

Without awareness, if you were uncomfortable, you would have remained so. Without discomfort, you had no reason to alter your position. *To change, you need to be both uncomfortable and aware of your discomfort.* Herein lies the rub. When you are in denial about your problems or rationalize that you're fine, you miss the *awareness* that is needed for change. Alternately, if your *discomfort* is so mild or slight that you barely notice it, you will have little motivation to change.

When I first meet my clients and students, I tell them that my job as a therapist and teacher is to make them uncomfortable, and that if I don't they should fire me. This often comes as a shock to clients who think I'm there solely to give them solace and make them feel better. It's true that making clients feel better is definitely my long-term goal, but I like to put it right out there at the beginning of treatment that they will not feel better until after they have felt worse, much worse. This is another way of saying that in order to find a new, healthier level of comfort, they will have to first increase their discomfort. (Not surprisingly, some people don't return after I give them this "bad" news.)

Am I saying that if you push yourself to nearly unbearable acts of discomfort, you will change more quickly? One might think so, but strangely enough the opposite is true. Too much discomfort becomes a major threat to oneself, and the mind is trained to drive it out of awareness, deconstructing the change equation. That means that we need to be judicious and compassionate with how much discomfort we try to bear. On the other hand, if our discomfort lacks sufficient intensity, it will not propel us forward. The proof is in the pudding: the only measure for determining whether you're allowing yourself to experience an adequate amount of discomfort (accompanied by your awareness of it) is whether your behavior actually changes.

What qualities promote behavioral change?

Heredity aside—and this is a large aside because the way we are genetically coded in terms of biochemistry and metabolism plays an integral part in determining how easy or hard it is to become a "normal" eater—your character traits will either facilitate or inhibit you from behavioral change. Previously I described two attitudes or perceptions that make change difficult, if not impossible: perfectionism and its dangerous cousin, all-or-nothing thinking. The less you think in failure-success terms and the more you recognize and value incremental change, the easier transforming your behavior will be.

Six personality traits are essential not only for changing your eating attitudes and behaviors, but for any kind of major personal or professional transformation. They are the three Cs and the three Ps: curiosity, compassion for self, caring for self, practice, patience, and persistence.

Curiosity means wondering about, rather than judging, what makes you do what you do. Judging yourself is like rushing down a dead-end street. It closes off the access to your mind and heart that you need for understanding your behavior. Curiosity, on the other hand, opens the doors of your mind and heart and gives you valuable information about your motivations and actions. Whenever you act or think in a way that troubles you, ask yourself, "I wonder why I did that?" or say, "That's interesting. Whatever was that all about?" Pretend you are Sherlock Holmes. The more clues you discover about your inner workings, the more quickly you will solve the mystery of what you need to do to change.

Compassion for self means never, ever saying something to yourself that you wouldn't say to a friend or young child. Why on earth would you call yourself names or speak ill of yourself in a way you would never think of doing to someone you love? This doesn't mean that you should avoid being honest with or even critical about yourself; you'll never transform yourself into a "normal" eater if you can't give yourself a fair and square appraisal. Compassion requires looking clearly at your faults and not thinking you are bad because of them. I know I'd prefer to be told that I'm doing something that isn't in my best interests with empathy and consideration rather than with cruelty and contempt. Who wouldn't?

Caring for self is so pivotal in working toward "normal" eating that it deserves far more than an explanatory paragraph. For that reason, it gets its own chapter (Chapter 8). For now, you can begin to think about four areas of self-care that you will need to work on to become a "normal" eater: physical, mental, emotional, and spiritual.

As for *practice*, remember that the more times the marble rolls down the groove in the sand, the deeper the groove will get. That's why practice makes progress (notice that I did *not* say perfect). The more you think or behave in a certain way, the more ingrained the pattern becomes. Neural pathways are reinforced every time you perform an action such as chewing slowly, stopping eating when you are no longer hungry, or walking right past the mirror without checking out your body. The more you do something, the easier it becomes, forming the positive feedback loop that promotes ultimate transformation.

Patience is something people say they either have or don't have, as if they were talking about owning a car or computer. But patience is not a commodity. It's a learned skill, albeit one that is influenced by our biochemistry, which helps to determine whether we tend to be mellow or easily frustrated. Patience basically involves sitting with the anxiety of wanting. Although this book will have a great deal more to say about anxiety when we consider how to tolerate feelings, for now let's just say that patience involves pacing yourself, lowering your expectations, and staying in the moment.

Just because you want something badly, even desperately, doesn't mean that you have to hurry up and get it. We humans are pretty clever, but we have not yet learned to speed up time. You will achieve your goals when you're ready and not a moment before. And you won't be ready to receive the gift of "normal" eating until you have cleaned out the mental and emotional space that's been occupied by compulsive, emotional, and restrictive eating.

Persistence is the ability to keep putting one foot in front of the other, no matter how frustrated or hopeless you feel. Persistence doesn't mean focusing exclusively on your goal 24/7; that's obsession. Persistence is knowing that it's OK and sometimes even necessary to take a rest from personal growth until you feel refreshed and energized and ready to move forward. But it also means you will not settle for less than whatever percentage of "normal" eating you've decided to aim for and that you'll keep going as long as you have appetite and breath!

If you possess most or many of the qualities I've just described, you'll find it easier to change your behaviors concerning food than if you don't. If you have few or none, you'll have to work on developing these attitudes and personality traits along with forging ahead to retrain yourself about food. Ironically, if you work hard enough to become a "normal" eater, it's highly likely that you will be creating an abundance of every one of these qualities: curiosity, compassion for self, care of self, practice, patience, and persistence.

How can I be sure I'll reach my goal of becoming a "normal" eater?

How can you ensure that you will reach any goal? First, by making certain that your goals are realistic, and second, by persevering until you reach them. Now we're back to *simple* versus *easy*. This is a simple formula, but in no way an easy one to follow. Remember when I said that moving from restrictive or compulsive/emotional eating toward "normal" eating may be the toughest challenge of your life? I meant it. The rewards that come from making peace with your eating problems feel nothing short of miraculous, but they have nothing whatsoever to do with miracles. The joys of having a healthier relationship with food come from years of incredibly hard work on yourself. If you want easy change, stop reading this book now, and return to it when you've come to terms with the fact that healing your eating problems will be ongoing, difficult, frustrating, nonlinear, and filled with intense soul-searching. That's the bad news.

The good news—that you'll reach your goals if you keep trying—can be illustrated by another simple exercise which requires you to be in a room where you can move around unselfconsciously. First, ask someone to be in the room with you for the purpose of standing by to help. Nothing bad will happen to you or them, I promise.

Stand up and pick a spot in the room to walk toward, along a path that has obstacles (say, a chair or TV, a desk or pile of papers). The spot should be far away but reachable. Now face your target and, as if you were measuring out carpet, place one foot directly in front of the other and walk toward your goal. Notice that you may need to walk around some things and crawl over or under others. You may even have to ask for help moving an object. That's fine. Just continue placing one foot immediately in front of the other, as if you're walking on a tightrope, until you reach your goal. Then stop. The exercise is complete.

What did you learn? I hope you concluded that obstacles don't have to get in your way to reach a goal. I suspect that in walking toward your target there were times when you were barreling full-steam ahead, times when you had to stop and think about how to correct your course, even times when you may have had to step backward or maneuver sideways to eventually end up moving forward. I hope that at least once you had to reach out for help. The point is that you kept moving and problem solving and getting help until you succeeded in reaching your goal.

In fact, the only way you could have failed to reach your objective was if you stopped putting one foot in front of the other. The same process works for becoming a "normal" eater. You may need to ask for help, creatively overcome obstacles on your own, and occasionally stop to take stock of your progress. There will be times when you feel as if you're zooming ahead and other times when success seems so far away that you want to give up. The only way you can fail is to stop trying. This is a theory not of psychology, but of physics: if you keep moving forward, you can't fail to get where you want to go.

This is probably a good time to think about your eating goal and how much of a "normal" eater you wish to be. Remember, a "normal" eater is someone who occasionally does at least some, if not all, of the following: makes impulsive and unsatisfying food choices, eats mindlessly, forgets to eat, lets herself get ravenous before eating, eats when she's not hungry, overeats or undereats, or makes other food-related bloopers. Like me, you may never be 100 percent a "normal" eater. Maybe your goal is 60 or 75 percent. This would be an excellent target. Just make sure that your "normal" eating goal is realistic for you in terms of genetics, eating and weight history, food allergies, metabolism, and biochemistry.

3

CHANGING BELIEFS, FEELINGS, AND BEHAVIORS

If I Start Now, Will I Finish Before I Die?

Now that you have a clearer understanding of how behavior changes, you may have realized that there's more to "normal" eating than merely following a set of rules having to do with hunger, craving, food choices, awareness, fullness, and satisfaction. In fact, you may think I'm crazy to imagine that you could so radically transform your eating attitudes and habits after years or decades of dysfunction. Sure, you might insist, a robot could be programmed to always follow the Rules of "Normal" Eating. But me? Never.

You would be both right and wrong. You're right that because you're a flesh-and-blood human being, you have thoughts, feelings, beliefs, attitudes, inclinations, desires, fears, and a general worldview that will influence your transformation into a "normal" eater. But you're wrong to underestimate yourself. It's because you *are* programmable that you *can* change. Part of the problem is that you've been programmed with the wrong instructions. This book will help you reprogram with the right ones.

How can I reprogram myself?

One excellent way is through Cognitive Therapy or Cognitive-Behavioral Therapy (CBT), which was pioneered by Albert Ellis and Aaron Beck in the 1960s. Mosby's *Medical, Nursing and Allied Health Dictionary* defines Cognitive Therapy as "any of the various methods of treating mental and emotional disorders that help a person change attitudes, perceptions, and patterns of thinking from irrational to realistic thoughts about self and situations."

In her book *Cognitive-Behavioral Therapy*, Paula Anne Ford-Martin defines CBT as "an action-oriented form of psychosocial therapy that assumes that maladaptive, or faulty, thinking patterns cause maladaptive behavior and 'negative emotions' . . . The treatment focuses on changing an individual's thoughts (cognitive patterns) in order to change his or her behavior and emotional state."

Below is the model that Cognitive-Behavioral Therapy uses to illustrate how beliefs, feelings, and behaviors interact.

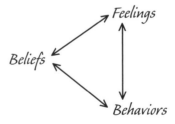

Simply put, your *beliefs*, whether conscious or unconscious, determine your *feelings* and *behaviors*. Change your beliefs, and your feelings and behaviors will be altered. Hold on to the same beliefs, and your feelings and behaviors will stay the same. Though beliefs generate feelings and behavior, the change process is not always linear. In fact, we often experience all three—believing, feeling, and behaving—nearly simultaneously, making it difficult to recognize that the belief actually came first.

For example, although you may sometimes take time to consider what foods you crave, you might often eat impulsively. Say you're sitting in a restaurant with a friend trying to relax after a stressful day at work or with the kids, and the waiter brings over a basket of piping hot rolls. Without thinking, you grab one and polish it off in a few quick bites. Maybe 60 seconds elapse between the moment you lay your eyes on the roll and that final swallow. You're probably aware of your *behavior* of eating the roll (but maybe not), and you may notice some *feelings* about having eaten it (relaxation, guilt, even surprise). You may even doubt that your beliefs had anything to do with what you did or felt. However, if you slowly dismantle this intricate cognitive-behavioral process, you'll see that all three reactions did not happen at exactly the same time. Your snap decision to grab a roll came *after* you decided it was OK to do so. Unfortunately, this decision was made outside your awareness.

Here's what happened behind the scenes. 1) You saw the roll. 2) Because you held the unconscious *belief* that food is a good reward after a stressful day, you *felt* you deserved the roll. 3) And your *behavior* was to eat it.

Just because you weren't aware that your belief prompted you to act doesn't mean it didn't. When it comes to making choices, your behavior and feelings are only the tip of the iceberg, while your beliefs make up the unseen base underneath. That's why you act automatically on beliefs, because they're buried so deeply that you don't even know they exist, leaving you disconnected from them. Your disconnection is the reason your behavior doesn't change even when you're working so hard to modify it.

Only when you are aware of and connected to your beliefs can you do anything about them. Change your beliefs, and new feelings and behaviors line up right behind them.

If your beliefs are unhealthy and dysfunctional, it follows that the behavior and feelings that are based on them will be dysfunctional too. Conversely, to develop healthy feelings and behaviors, you must first have healthy, functional beliefs.

To become a "normal" eater, then, you must build a belief system that promotes "normal" eating and think about food as "normal" eaters do. Changes in your feelings and behaviors concerning food will come as a direct result of revamping your beliefs. For example, if you *believe* as a restrictive eater that escarole is a better choice of food than an éclair, then you will choose (*behavior*) the escarole. This behavior may leave you *feeling* deprived. On the other hand, if you *believe* as a compulsive/emotional eater that the éclair far outweighs (no pun intended) the escarole, you'll go for (*behavior*) the éclair, which may leave you *feeling* guilty.

If you're a "normal" eater, you will *believe* that food has well-documented nutritional value but no intrinsic universal or absolute appeal. You'll select (*behavior*) the escarole or the éclair depending on what you feel like eating. You will *feel* nothing either way about the moral merit of your decision, although you may have feelings about the food itself—distaste that the éclair is too sweet or delight that it is absolutely scrumptious; pleasure that the escarole is crisp and fresh, or disappointment that it is wilted and bitter.

Why do we need beliefs?

In the next chapter we'll explore the food and eating beliefs held by restrictive, emotional/compulsive, and "normal" eaters. But first let's look at how and why beliefs originate. Along with other kinds of learning, beliefs take root at an unconscious level early in life without your even knowing it. Beliefs settle silently into your mind and, for the most part, exist far below consciousness. We all have beliefs—predictable, patterned ways of viewing ourselves and the world. Without them, life would be unbearably chaotic and frightening because:

- Beliefs help us make sense of and give meaning to the world. (Examples: I must have gotten sick because I kissed my aunt who had the flu. My friend is late because she can never get off the phone with her son. If I work hard I will succeed.)

- Beliefs help orient us in the context of time and space. (Examples: The sun is up, so it must be morning. Spring follows winter.)

- Beliefs give us a sense of internal stability and familiarity and provide a way to navigate through life with a modicum of safety and security. (Examples: I am a whiz with numbers. I know how to change a tire. If I take an umbrella, I won't get wet. If I get too close to people, I'll get hurt.)

Imagine not having beliefs! You wouldn't know what to make of anything that goes on inside or outside yourself. Life would be a series of helter-skelter, unpredictable, random acts, a string of unconnected dots. Instead of thinking, "The sidewalk is slippery and so I'd better proceed with caution," you might view the two ideas as unrelated and be shocked when you end up on your fanny. Lacking a way of interpreting the world aimed at promoting safety and reducing harm, your thoughts, actions, and feelings would come as a total surprise. Beliefs are similar to memory, in that they form a link between events and sensations and help you predict and anticipate the future.

On my birthday, I expect to receive cards from friends and family because they have sent them before and because this is the norm in our society. This rational belief is based on my experience. Of course, I may also have the irrational belief that "When it's my birthday, everyone I know *should* send me cards." Then I will feel disappointed when they don't. Notice how the *feeling* of disappointment follows the *belief*. If I were to extend this example to include a *behavior*, I might end up not sending a card to Uncle Joe on his birthday simply because he didn't send one to me. I might call my friend Denise and chew her out for forgetting my special day. The progression would go as follows: 1) My *belief* that everyone I know should send cards on my birthday leads to 2) my *feeling* disappointed when they don't, which leads to 3) my not sending them a card (*behavior*) on their birthday or chewing them out.

Where do beliefs come from?

As I said before, beliefs are formed unconsciously in childhood to make meaning of the world. You couldn't stop yourself from forming beliefs if you tried. It would be as impossible as willing your heart to stop beating. As a child, you internalized beliefs from your parents and other caretakers when they advised, suggested, or implied what you should think about things such as religion, morality, politics, and your own value. Their expectations taught you what they thought was right and wrong and formed the basis of your unconscious belief system.

As you grew older, you incorporated beliefs from other sources—teachers, neighbors, friends, relatives, the media, the general culture. You also learned from your own experience, which either reinforced or challenged your original beliefs.

Parents who have a rigid belief system often insist that their children share the same beliefs they hold. As a child, you had little choice but to agree or act as if you agreed. For example, if your father believed it was wrong to waste food, he may have sat at the table with you until you finished all your food, as my father did more times than I care to remember. By his actions and words, my father let me know that he would think poorly of me unless I was a member of the clean-plate club. He never threatened punishment; he didn't have to because I wanted so very much to please him. Not surprisingly, I adopted his belief and grew into an adult who believed it was wrong to waste food. Also—no surprise—when I attempted to change this belief, it was hard to shake the feeling that I was doing something very bad and wrong, even though my father had been dead more than 20 years. As you can see, beliefs are made of powerful stuff.

Another way you learn beliefs is by observing what your parents do. Even if my father hadn't said a word to me about finishing my food, if he never left a morsel on his own plate, I would naturally conclude that it was wrong to do so. Parents model behavior, showing us how to do things. Your parents, of course, don't necessarily realize that they're modeling behavior. My father probably thought he was merely finishing his dinner! But between watching him clean his plate (and sometimes everyone else's!) at every meal, and having him sit with me until mine was shiny as a mirror, I got the point—never, ever waste food. And over time this message turned into the belief that I was bad if I did.

If you take the time, you can retrace your most basic beliefs, the ones that form the bedrock of your feelings and behaviors, to understand how they evolved from your upbringing. These beliefs include assumptions about such things as trusting people, asking for and receiving help, how scary or safe the world is, your value as a human being, and whether you are a powerless victim or an empowered individual. Remember that beliefs are not merely the words your parents tell you; they are the unwritten (and often unconscious) instructions about how you should live your life.

Take learning about honesty, for example. A belief that you should always try to be honest evolves from a combination of your parents' direct instruction ("It's wrong to be dishonest"), their indirect expression (disappointed faces when you lied), and modeling (watching a parent return a dropped wallet to a stranger). After years of similar experiences on the subject, you absorbed the message that honesty is the best policy, which became part of your belief system.

Do all beliefs make sense?

Cognitive therapy maintains that there are two kinds of beliefs or types of thinking: irrational and rational. As described in *A New Guide to Rational Living* by Albert Ellis, Ph.D. and Robert Harper, Ph.D., quoting Dr. Maxie Maultsby, "Rational thinking has the following four characteristics: 1) It [bases itself] primarily on objective fact as opposed to subjective opinion. 2) If acted upon, it most likely will result in the preservation of your life and limb rather than your premature death or injury. 3) If acted upon, it produces your personally defined life's goals most quickly. 4) If acted upon, it prevents undesirable personal and/or environmental conflict."

Maultsby is saying that <u>rational thinking is life-enhancing and supports healthy goals by promoting healthy feelings and behaviors</u>. Irrational thinking is life-threatening and leads you in directions that will ultimately cause mental, emotional, and even physical harm. Let's return to my earlier example of having learned to finish the food on my plate and see how my belief that "It's wrong to waste food" stacks up against Maultsby's criteria for rational thinking. You can decide if my belief is rational or not.

- *First, is my belief based on fact, and if so, what is the objective evidence that wasting food is wrong?* There is not a shred of objective evidence here regarding causation, that leaving a french fry on my plate is criminal, sinful, or of harm to anyone. But there is proof aplenty that it isn't healthy for me to continue eating when I'm full.

- *Second, by not wasting food and finishing everything on my plate, will my health be enhanced and my life lengthened?* Hardly. In fact, the opposite is true. By consistently eating when I'm not hungry, I take the chance of becoming morbidly obese, which is a health risk. As important, by finishing all the food on my plate, I'm reinforcing a disconnect from my body rather than validating that only I know how much food to take in.

- *Third, will finishing all my food help me reach my life's goals quickly?* It certainly won't, if one of my goals is to be a healthy "normal" eater.

- *Fourth, will becoming a member of the clean-plate club prevent undesirable personal and/or environmental conflict?* On the contrary, I'll feel more conflicted if I polish off my food because I'll be going against my body's clear signals of fullness.

Of course, if I were living, say, in Somalia or anywhere that was suffering a food shortage, my belief about not wasting food would be very rational. By finishing all the food on my plate, I would be ensuring good health and a long life. This example shows that the validity of beliefs, including whether they are rational or irrational, depends on context. You could even say that my belief about scraping my plate clean was rational when I was a child because I needed my father's approval in order to remain emotionally and physically healthy, that is, to survive. The belief became irrational when I was no longer dependent on my father to feed and take care of me and when his approval no longer mattered in terms of my survival.

You can take any belief and measure it against Maultsby's criteria to see if it's rational or irrational. Maultsby's criteria work as well for political and professional beliefs as they do for personal ones. The more frequently you evaluate your beliefs to see if they are rational or irrational, the easier the process will get. Remember, your beliefs should improve your life and support your long-term goals.

Can I really rid myself of irrational beliefs and replace them with rational ones?

Creating a life based on rational beliefs is like winning in the game of Scrabble®. The more usable letter tiles you have on your rack and the fewer turkeys, the more high-point words you can create. The higher your word score each turn, the more likely you'll win the game. Similarly, if you have a functional set of beliefs to steer you through life, you will be able to make healthy choices. Each time you make a healthy choice, you are scoring points toward a winning life.

So what do you do if, after studying the Scrabble board intently, you look at your tiles and realize there is no way your Z, Q, and two Vs are going to configure into any kind of word? Well, you can opt for a total trade and dump the lot, selecting a whole new set of tiles to play with. Or you can keep your most usable tiles and swap the least usable ones. Of course, without peeking at your new tiles first, there's no guarantee that they will be any better than the old ones. But if you couldn't make any words before, you have little to lose and much to gain by dumping the lot of them. By the same token, if your life isn't working with your current beliefs, what do you have to lose by trying out some new ones?

Unlike Scrabble tiles, you *can* take a peek at beliefs before making them your own. Indeed, you must. Pretend you're taking them on an imaginary test drive to determine if they'll get you where you want to go. Play out the feelings and behaviors that will evolve from a new belief, and see if they match up with your life goals.

An even better belief analogy is what I call the Belief Store. I took the idea from my love of consignment-store shopping—in I go with my old, boring clothes, and out I come with something new and exciting, at least to me. My Belief Store is as huge as 100 airplane hangars, and it contains every rational belief imaginable, and then some. Each aisle is clearly marked to indicate what kind of belief it contains, with categories and subcategories— religion, appearance, politics, guns, abortion, weight, food, art, music, self-esteem, sex, child rearing, war, etc. All you have to do is bring in the old, irrational beliefs you want to get rid of, then take your time strolling up and down the aisles checking out all the new rational beliefs that are available. There are endless racks of possibilities to choose from, and you can try them on to see if they feel right. If they don't, you can keep looking until you find the precise beliefs that suit you. There's even a customer service desk with a therapist who can steer you in the right direction. If you can't find just what you want on the racks, she'll help tailor beliefs that will fit you to a T.

What are you waiting for? If you know you have beliefs that aren't working for you, bundle them up and trot them over to the Belief Store. Remember, you'll be getting a three-for-one deal because when you transform your beliefs, your feelings and behavior will also change for the better.

Can I change my feelings before my beliefs?

Although changing your beliefs is essential for becoming a "normal" eater and will facilitate your transformation, you can also work from the other two points on the cognitive-behavioral triangle: feelings and behavior. Because feelings are so powerful, you may find it difficult to try to change them before your beliefs, but the job is far from impossible. Of course, it depends on what you believe about your ability to alter your feelings! If you believe that *you* are in charge of *them*, you'll be able to shift out of uncomfortable feelings states more easily. If you believe that feelings rule you and that's the end of that (or, even more irrationally, that others can *make* you have certain feelings), you'll succumb to whatever you're feeling with hopelessness, helplessness, and, perhaps, even despair.

Here's an exercise that can prove to you that you have the ability to change your feelings. Think of a time when you were sad or disappointed. It may be a recent or distant memory. The exercise works best if you don't pick a memory that packs too big a punch; choose one that has some intensity but is not overwhelming. Now try to conjure up all the details of the context in which the feeling arose—your age, the setting, the people involved, the incident or situation that caused the feelings. Let yourself sink into the emotional discomfort and sit with it for a few minutes, stoking the fires of your distress until you're reliving the experience.

Now change gears and consciously force yourself to come up with a memory that makes you downright joyful, lifts your spirits, takes you right over the top. At first it will be hard to let go of the sadness or disappointment, but continue to try to shift your mood to a lighter, more upbeat one by focusing exclusively on the joyful memory. Again, attend to the details of the context that produced your exhilaration. Let it flow through your body like white light for a few minutes, feeding your delight with more particulars if it starts to ebb. Notice how your entire body feels better, lighter, brighter, as you absorb all the joy and expand into it, and how your energy increases and your outlook brightens.

Once again, now, switch gears: let go of the joyful feeling and return to the memory that evoked your initial sadness or disappointment. Stir up the embers of the memory until it sears your heart and allow yourself to be consumed by the pain. Notice the changes in your body, how energy seeps out, how dark and maybe even scary the world seems, how utterly helpless you feel. Then, for the final time, let go of the emotional pain and again shift your attention to your joyful memory. Extract every bit of happiness from the memory until you are positively gushing with pleasure.

I hope you were able to shift from one emotional state to another, showing yourself that you *can* control your feelings. If you were unable to rise above your unhappiness, it may mean either that the emotion was too intense or that you irrationally believed that you couldn't make the shift. Moreover, such is the nature of emotions that misery will keep trying to worm its weasely way into a happy heart. But that hardly means you have to let it. By practicing this exercise, you'll improve at shifting emotions, so that when you need to pull yourself up and out of your misery, you'll have more muscle and increased leverage.

Can you guess what bearing this exercise has on your behavior and beliefs? It proves that if you change your feelings, your behavior is likely to change along with it. For example, when you feel sad or disappointed, your body often responds with fatigue and heaviness. You want nothing more than to crawl into bed (or drag your sorry self toward the kitchen). But when you're joyful, you're practically bursting with energy and can think of a million fun things to do. These are examples of how your behavior follows your feelings.

Changing your feelings also has the power to shift your beliefs. If you notice what you are thinking when you feel sad or disappointed, you will probably come up with negative beliefs such as *This is awful. I can't bear the pain. I screwed up again. Why do terrible things always happen to me?* If you notice what you were thinking when you feel joyful, you will likely find yourself in a positive mental state, believing *Aren't I lucky? I've sure got what it takes! Gee, isn't life grand!* Your beliefs align with your feelings.

How about changing my behavior first?

Give it a whirl. Try this experiment and see what happens. Take a 10-minute walk around your neighborhood. If you live in an isolated area, go to a spot that's crowded with people, such as a mall or supermarket.

For the first 5 minutes of the exercise, skulk along with your head down. Scowl, frown, and avoid eye contact with people. Notice their reactions. They'll likely scowl back or avert their gaze. Pay attention to how you feel in response to their reactions. Kind of sour, I bet. For the second 5 minutes, take on a completely different persona. Make eye contact with and smile at every person you see. Say hello, wink or nod. You'll be surprised at how many people grin back or say something cheerful. And you'll be surprised how good that makes you feel.

Observe the progression. When you change your behavior from negative to positive, you receive a parallel positive reaction from people, and you feel better! What goes around comes around. Changes in behavior lead to changes in feelings. The same shift happens when you're feeling grumpy and you push yourself to call a good friend, jump on the treadmill, listen to your favorite CD, or do something nice for someone. Your feelings grow more positive, and you think differently. You go from thinking *Life sure is hard/awful/frustrating/not much fun/a struggle* to *Things aren't so bad. I can get through this. I'm going to make it.* Changes in behavior lead to changes in feelings, which lead to changes in beliefs.

Here's one more example of how this works. Let's say you have a belief that people are generally disrespectful to you. You're easily injured, and out of your hurt, you treat other people with little regard. They respond in kind, which reinforces your belief that they're disrespectful. The cycle is an endless, negative loop, a boomerang that, unfortunately, does come back—to knock you down!

So, let's change the outcome by first changing the feeling, then changing the behavior. Let's go with your belief that people are disrespectful to you. That doesn't mean you have to *feel* disrespected. You could decide that they're rude morons or that they're having a bad day. Moreover, you could decide that even though they're inconsiderate of you, you'll behave nicely toward them. If they're kind and polite in return, it might just change your belief that people are generally disrespectful. In fact, you could feel bent out of shape when people are rude to you and still decide to behave kindly toward them, proving to yourself that you can rise above your feelings. Again, there's a good chance that they will, in turn, be kinder to you, which will make you feel better and transform your thinking.

Please don't just take my word that you have the power to change your beliefs, feelings, and behavior and that by altering one corner of the cognitive-behavioral triangle, you can powerfully influence the other two. Instead, experiment. Purposely act differently than you usually do (change your *behavior*), and check out people's reactions—and your reactions to their reactions (changing your *feeling*). Notice if your new emotional response alters your take on the situation (changes your *belief*).

Or, try out a different attitude (change your *feeling*) in a situation, and see how it affects what you do (changes your *behavior*). Then see if *doing* something different challenges your assumptions (changes your *beliefs*). The greater your understanding of the intricate connections among beliefs, feelings, and behaviors, the easier it will be to transform yourself from a restrictive or compulsive/emotional eater into a "normal" one.

I hope you realize by now that it's your irrational belief about your lack of power that keeps you stuck in the first place—with food, weight, and body image issues. The power to change is inside you, itching to get out. Dare to unleash it and watch your life transform itself. Dare to believe.

4

IRRATIONAL BELIEFS ABOUT FOOD, EATING, WEIGHT, AND BODY

You Mean My Beliefs Are Supposed to Make Sense?

I hope you're rapidly gaining insight into how your beliefs, feelings, and behaviors are all connected, and that you're developing a deeper appreciation for the hard work involved in reaching your "normal" eating goals. Imagine that your belief system acts as the engine that runs your mental machinery, causing you to feel what you feel and do what you do. Of course, your biochemistry also plays a significant and sometimes overriding, though hidden, role in this complicated process by intricately regulating your moods and energy flow on a cellular level. But, for the purpose of understanding how to become a "normal" eater, think of your belief system as the generator that drives your feelings and behaviors. If the generator isn't working properly, its output—your behaviors and feelings—will be substandard and ineffective. Tune up or replace the generator, and watch the quality of your life improve!

When are you going to get to the point and tell me what "normal" eaters believe?

Soon. I understand your impatience, but you're putting the cart before the horse. First you have to recognize what *you*, as an emotional/compulsive or restrictive eater, currently believe. After you've explored those beliefs, you'll know exactly what "normal" eaters believe: the opposite!

I've never met a person with disordered eating who didn't long for instant change (including me, way back when!). And who could blame them? That's why you love quick-fix diets. You're impatient to know everything about becoming a "normal" eater right away so you can hurry up and get your eating right. You want to be there already. Is it possible that your impatience is part of the problem and that it might even get in the way of becoming a "normal" eater and a healthier person?

Relax, be patient, slow yourself down. You're not making instant pudding here; you are not microwavable! You're trying to transform deeply ingrained, decades-old beliefs, feelings, and behaviors that are painfully familiar, second nature, so much a part of you that you may rarely notice them. Think *slow cooker* and imagine yourself as a stew simmering over low heat until all the ingredients blend together and the taste is perfect. If you turn up the heat too quickly, your stew will burn. And that's what will happen if you try to whip yourself into a "normal" eater overnight: you'll burn yourself out. So start with the belief that change will come if you keep working at it—and it will.

What are examples of irrational beliefs?

Rather than have you waste precious mental energy reinventing the wheel, I've compiled a list of the major beliefs—irrational, of course—held by restrictive and compulsive/emotional eaters. Some of these beliefs apply only to undereating or overeating, but most hold true for anyone with food problems.

The list is far from exhaustive and may not cover every irrational thought you have about food, eating, weight, and your body. For now, just notice which beliefs resonate and express your disordered thinking. If you realize that something you believe is missing, jot it down. Soon you'll learn how to identify your own irrational beliefs so you'll have a comprehensive, personal list.

1. Irrational Beliefs About Food

- There are good foods (that is, low-calorie, low-fat) and bad foods (that is, high-calorie, high-fat).
- Food is the enemy.
- Food is dangerous and scary.
- Food is scarce.
- Food will make me fat.
- Food takes care of me.
- Food is love and comfort.
- I need to be in tight control around food.
- Food should never, ever, under penalty of death—or worse—be wasted.

- I can never get enough food.
- I should eat only foods that are nutritious.
- I'll never learn to feel satisfied with food.
- I should never eat fattening foods.
- Food will solve all my problems.
- Eating low-cal food has to rule my life or I'll be as big as a horse.
- If food is on my plate, I have to finish it.
- Food is my best friend.
- Food is a good reward.
- Food is my life.

2. Irrational Beliefs About Eating

- I have to eat fast or someone else will get more than I do.
- Eating will make me fat.
- If I don't think about what I'm eating, it can't hurt me or put pounds on me.
- Eating is a painful process I wish I could do without.
- It's better to not eat and be thin than to be fat.
- I can't think about eating without becoming anxious.
- If I start eating something I like, I'll never stop.
- Eating is better than feeling emotional pain or discomfort.
- I can't stand eating around other people.
- Overeating is always a bad thing, and "normal" eaters never overeat.
- I'm ashamed of how I eat.

- I never know what to eat.
- I should always know what I want to eat.
- Hunger is scary.
- I can't let myself feel hungry.
- I should eat what other people want me to eat or what others are eating.
- If I get together with people, eating has to be involved.
- My eating behaviors are so shameful, I can't let anyone see them.
- Eating fills the emptiness inside me.
- Eating is the only pleasure I have in life.
- Feeling good or bad about myself depends on what I eat or don't eat.
- Denying myself food shows I'm in control of my eating and, therefore, deprivation and restriction equal emotional strength.
- If I can't find exactly what I want to eat, I feel deprived.

3. Irrational Beliefs About Weight

- I have to be thin.
- Thin equals a happy, successful, perfect life.
- I won't be happy with myself unless I lose weight.
- Fat equals miserable, unhappy, and not deserving of or enjoying a good life.
- I should weigh myself every day.
- I should never weigh myself.

- If I didn't weigh myself, I wouldn't know what to eat.
- Because people only see my fat body, I don't need to bother about my appearance.
- Being fat gets in the way of all the good things I want in life.
- Thin is more lovable than fat.
- I should weigh what the magazines and weight charts say I should.
- Thin people are lucky and can eat whatever they want.
- Large people should only eat low-calorie, low-fat foods.
- The only way for me to be happy is to be or stay thin.
- I'm too fat.
- Looking good is more important than being happy inside myself.
- A person can never be too thin.
- Feeling proud or ashamed of myself depends on what I weigh.
- No accomplishment of mine is as important as being or becoming a thin person.
- It's too scary to gain weight, even a pound.
- If I gain a pound or two, who knows when I'll stop gaining weight?

4. Irrational Beliefs About My Body

- I'll never be happy with my body.
- My body should be perfect.
- I can't trust my body to give itself the good care it needs.

- I can't trust my body to feed itself in a way that keeps me healthy and satisfied.
☆ - My body is something to be ashamed of.
- I can't love myself while I'm fat.
- I can only love myself while I'm thin.
- The purpose of a body is to look good.
☆ - I'll never be proud of my body.
- The only thing I am proud of is my body.
- I'm not in control of my body.
- If I can focus on controlling my body, I can avoid looking at my mess of a life.
☆ - My body will never learn when to say yes and no to food at the right times and in the right amounts.
- What other people think about my body is more important than what I think about it.
☆ - No one will ever love me if I'm fat.

I hope that you found at least a few beliefs in each of the four categories that ring true for you. If acknowledging these beliefs has led to your feeling badly about yourself, see if you can gently push away the judgment. Remember, one of the key tenets of transformation to "normal" eating is to replace judgment with curiosity and compassion. Before moving on, try to maneuver your attitude into one of nonjudgment and genuine interest in why you think as you do. Become a detective, not an officer of the courts!

Notice the common themes that run through these irrational beliefs—the repetition of words such as *always*, *never*, *enemy*, *dangerous*, *scarce*, *scared*, *can't*, and *should*; the tone of blame, negativity, and hopelessness; the intense rigidity of all-or-nothing thinking; the shame and denial of pleasure; the off-with-her-head kinds of judgments. In short, the irrational thinking! Try reading the list again without judgment. Holding some of these beliefs doesn't make you a bad person. If you feel bad when one of the beliefs hits home, remind yourself that beliefs can be changed and that you're in the process of changing them.

How do I identify exactly what I believe about food, eating, weight, and my body?

In cognitive-behavioral language, identifying a belief is called *framing* it. Framing a belief means describing or explaining it. Here are some helpful hints for framing or identifying beliefs:

- Use the three "S's"—keep them short, simple, and straightforward. Don't try to embellish or cram a number of ideas into one belief.

- Use present tense, active verbs such as *like*, *dislike*, *desire*, *wish*, *is*, and *are*.

- If possible, state them in the positive, not the negative, which means eliminating words such as *isn't*, *aren't*, *won't*, *can't*, and *shouldn't*.

Think of framing beliefs as you would choosing colors to paint a room. Would you go into a paint store and ask the clerk for two gallons of yellow? I doubt it. More likely you'd try to be as specific as possible and ask for pale gold, sunburst yellow, or daffodil. In the same way that certain colors leap out at you when you're flipping through a paint chart, you'll recognize when a belief hits home. And just as you might have to go through a slew of paint chips to find the exact color that suits you, you will have to put a substantial amount of time into accurately identifying your beliefs.

Some of your beliefs will be in the form of "I" statements, such as "I will never learn to eat normally" or "I am only lovable when I'm thin." Others will be more general, such as "People who pig out are disgusting," or "There are 'good' and 'bad' foods." The fact that the beliefs are constructed as personal or general statements isn't important. What is crucial is *nailing the belief exactly as you think it.* That means listening very hard to what your inner voice is telling you. If you can't hear it, then you may need to be very quiet and turn up the volume. Don't give up; keep listening and it will come.

Don't worry if you generate a number of beliefs that sound similar. For example, "I should finish all the food on my plate" is not precisely the same as "I should never waste food." They are pretty close, but not identical. The point of identifying beliefs is to produce as many as you can, so that you know that all your cognitive bases are covered. If you try to lump similar beliefs together, you may end up with a watered-down version of your belief system and miss vital information about what you really think.

Now it's time to make your own list. Feel free to use my list as a basis and to tweak any belief that doesn't fit you quite right. Make sure that you also do some independent, creative thinking. Here's how. Get pencil and paper and quickly write down as many beliefs as you can about eating, food, weight, and body. Don't let your pen leave the paper, and keep writing until your brain goes blank. Just go on churning out those beliefs, no matter how awkward or silly or scary they sound.

When you're done, take a moment to scour the crevices of your mind where hidden irrational beliefs might be lurking. Wait a few minutes to see if you can discover additional beliefs. If not, review your list and work with each and every belief to make it a mirror image of what you believe. This is a time to be a real fussbudget. You want to craft each belief to match your exact thinking. Keep the list handy as you read this book and go through the day, so you can add beliefs that seem relevant. Each belief you uncover is one more opportunity to change your thinking.

Do all overeaters or undereaters share the same irrational beliefs?

Because both restrictive and emotional/compulsive eaters fear food and have an unhealthy relationship with it, they naturally have a great many irrational ideas in common. Here are some of the ways they think (and, therefore, feel) similarly.

- They don't trust their bodies.
- They lack healthy internal controls around food.
- They view food as something other than fuel and pleasure.
- They generally feel helpless and anxious around food.
- They have questions about what is enough.
- They give food a much larger place in life than "normal" eaters do.
- They are disconnected from their body's natural mechanisms for feeling comfortable around and enjoying food.
- They suffer shame when they don't eat according to how they feel they should.
- They focus on food and use food to manage uncomfortable feelings.
- They lack a repertoire of healthy self-care approaches.

Plaguing both kinds of eaters are questions about what they deserve in life, the way they're managing their lives, and how they can get their emotional needs met effectively.

While compulsive overeaters consciously or unconsciously believe they can't stop eating, compulsive undereaters believe they shouldn't start. While overeaters believe there's never enough food to satisfy them, undereaters derive little joy from food and rarely feel satisfied. While emotional eaters head for food when they are upset, restrictive eaters deny themselves the foods they want.

Compulsive eaters believe that food is their best friend and has magical emotional healing powers, that they can never get enough food and can't stop eating once they start, that they deserve to eat as a reward, that saying no to food is scary and unsatisfying. Compulsive noneaters, on the other hand, believe that almost any amount of food is too much, that they don't deserve to nourish themselves, that saying yes to food is scary, and that the act of not eating has magical healing powers.

However, because each eater's history is unique, beliefs may vary to some degree. Some binge eaters believe that gorging themselves on vegetables and rice cakes is acceptable because these foods are "healthy" (read "good"), while others will snarf up anything that isn't likely to kill them on the spot. Some restrictive eaters believe that swallowing one calorie of anything over their preestablished daily limit qualifies as a felony, while others believe the only true sin is to relish foods they crave and adore.

When it comes to belief systems, the widest gulf is not between restrictive and emotional/compulsive eaters but between disordered and "normal" eaters. In fact, the gulf is so wide you could drive a fleet of Good Humor® trucks right through it! Not surprisingly, the beliefs of "normal" eaters are the antithesis, the exact mirror image, of the beliefs of restrictive and compulsive/emotional eaters. *Which means that whether you are a chronic overeater, a restrictive eater, or a combination of both, you will need to do a 180 with your beliefs to become a "normal" eater.*

This may come as shocking or disheartening news, but it's important that you realize what's in store before you start working on assessing and changing your beliefs. Most likely, to heal yourself you'll have to turn your belief system about food, eating, weight and your body (along with many core cognitions) inside out. You'll have to give your belief system a rough shake as you would a tree full of apples, so that the rotten beliefs will fall off and die, and the tree can grow new, healthy fruit.

Is the chatter in my head related to my irrational beliefs?

The chatter in your head *is* your irrational beliefs, in this case your beliefs about food, eating, weight, and your body, elbowing themselves into your mind. Also called negative self-talk, chatter often originates in the external world of family and friends, culture and the media, and seeps into your unconscious. It's nothing but your busy mind's misguided attempt to keep you out of harm's way by telling you what's right for you. Although the goal is honorable—to prevent you from making mistakes in life and failing—the methodology is flawed because chatter is rigid and simplistic, out of touch with your current internal and external reality, and based on preconceived (often ill-conceived) notions.

The authoritative voice in your head that drones just below your radar is chatter. You kind of hear it and kind of don't. Chatter has nothing to do with veracity, fact, or what's right for you; it's your distorted thinking masquerading as truth. You can generally identify chatter by its rigid, judgmental quality and limited vocabulary. Chatter usually starts with, "I should, shouldn't, can't, must, mustn't, have to, need to, ought not, or ought to." It often throws in a misleading take on how you behave, as in, "I always" or "I never," that rarely can be backed up by evidence.

Chatter is all brakes and no accelerator. It prevents you from taking risks, acting in new ways, and generally moving your life forward. It sneaks in unwanted editorial comments about everything you think, feel, and do. Here's some typical eating- and weight-related chatter:

- You need to go on a diet.
- You must gobble up that last slice of pumpkin pie this instant.
- There's no possible way you can throw out the rest of that linguini.
- Eating whatever your body wants means you're out of control.
- The less you eat, the better you'll feel.
- You'll never make it past the donut shop.
- You'd better eat now because it's lunchtime.
- You're too old to start exercising.
- You have to say yes when you're offered food.
- Trumping your appetite means you're a strong person.
- You're too fat or thin to care about clothes.
- You'll die if you put on a pound.

- You'll never get to the weight you want and stay there.
- You can't possibly become a "normal" eater.
- You shouldn't be hungry.
- Forget about food.
- You'll never be able to trust your body.
- You're too fat.

Chatter comes in a variety of clever disguises designed to slip by undetected: the nutrition expert, instructing you to munch a carrot because you need vitamin A instead of the brownie with the gooey frosting you love; your mother's gentle reminder to order something light and eat like a lady when you're on a date; the food police, threatening untold punishment if you dare to eat the sweets and treats you crave; your child self, whining and whimpering for (or demanding) an ice-cream cone; the martyr, suffering and denying yourself pleasure; the victim, moping because there's nothing to do but eat; the attention seeker, clinging to feeling special by being thin; your father, insisting that you clean your plate because he works hard to keep you well fed; the religious zealot, admonishing you that it's a sin to enjoy or waste food; the ascetic, commanding you to refuse to succumb to hunger; your grandmother, consoling you with goodies when you're feeling sick or blue; the caretaker, making sure everyone else is fed; the rebel, proving by starving or stuffing yourself that you know better than everyone else; the magician, tricking you into believing that what you do with food has no consequences.

Unless you're determined, single-minded, and persistent, chatter, like head lice, is difficult to get rid of. However, it can often be short-circuited by a few challenging questions:

- Why shouldn't I?
- How come I need to?
- Who says I must always or never?

By confronting chatter as soon as it begins, you can avoid letting it drone on and on until it infects your thoughts, feelings, and behavior.

To identify chatter in the early stages of becoming a "normal" eater, it pays to be suspicious of all your familiar thoughts about food, eating, weight, and your body, as well as any beliefs that sound clichéd and canned. Watch out for thinking that's hard and fast, rigid, extreme, or simplistic. Be wary whenever a thought is annoyingly intrusive and full of its own importance, then deflates under minimal scrutiny.

Here are some ways to turn off chatter. When you hear yourself saying things that run counter to "normal" eating or to feeling accepting of your body, write them down. Keep a chatter list and read it once in a while to remind yourself what your own particular brand of nonsense-thinking sounds like. When you get a blast of chatter, step up to the plate and challenge it. Remember that chatter is nothing more than your irrational beliefs on speakerphone. Take each line of chatter and replace it with a rational thought or belief. Proclaim the new belief loudly and proudly.

When you become more used to recognizing the noise in your head, it'll be easier to identify chatter and chase it away. Remember, the only voice you ever want to hear is one that speaks your own rational truth. No matter what anyone has ever told you or what you've ever believed about yourself, only you have the answers that will guide you toward "normal" eating.

It's tempting to listen to other voices—inside your head and outside—because if you follow their advice and it's wrong, you can argue that you're not responsible for making a mistake. But you don't build confidence or a store of your own wisdom by listening to someone else. The only way you'll grow truly wise is to tune in to your inner voice, then either fail and learn from your mistake, or succeed and build your belief in yourself. So listen for that internal voice that supports your health and welfare; that comes from a place of abundance, generosity, compassion, and good will; that's imbued with reason, intelligence, logic, and insight; and that has your best long-term interests in mind.

Change is a challenge

Giving up irrational thinking and a lifelong twisted obsession with food is not for the faint of heart. You cannot merely tweak your beliefs about calories and forbidden foods and suddenly awake the next morning a model "normal" eater. At the risk of sounding corny, the depth and scope of this process might leave you feeling as if you have more on your plate than you can handle. It *is* hard, hard work to unlearn decades of unhealthy thinking and habits and then develop and relearn healthy replacements; it takes the courage of a lion, the ferocity of a bear, and the patience of a saint!

But the rewards are like none other: freeing yourself from the yoke of obsession and compulsion; feeling healthy and normal around food; knowing that at long last you can take care of yourself inside and out and that no one will ever be able to snatch that ability away from you; and creating a life that is truly satisfying and fulfilling, a life you would never have had if you had continued your unhealthy love affair with food.

Letting go of a dead-end, destructive relationship with food gives you the chance of a lifetime to find true love, the greatest love of all, which is love of self. Believe me, there's nothing finer. In the next chapter you'll learn how to turn the irrational beliefs that keep you stuck in a negative eating pattern into rational beliefs that are the foundation of "normal" eating.

5

BELIEFS OF "NORMAL" EATERS

May I Have a Belief Implant, Please?

The beliefs of disordered and "normal" eaters run on two parallel tracks, and no matter how far you follow them down the line, never the twain shall meet. If you want an improved relationship with food, you need to jump off your dead-end track, cross over, and hop onto the track marked "normal" eating. You may remember from Chapter 3 that it is possible to rehab your belief system by changing your behaviors or feelings. Cognitive change *can* happen this way, but the approach is rather haphazard, like uprooting one garden weed at a time, then planting a single flower in its place. Using this slapdash method, it would take an awfully long time to transform your yard from a tangle of weeds to a luscious garden.

A more effective plan would be to grab a shovel and, sweating and grunting, turn over every inch of yard to uproot your weeds and plant your flowers all in one fell swoop. Now *that's* an efficient use of time and energy. Think of irrational beliefs as the weeds you want to remove from your garden, and think of rational, "normal" eating beliefs as the flowers you want to plant in their stead.

In Chapter 4 we discussed *framing* or identifying your beliefs. In cognitive-behavioral terms, a belief makeover is called *reframing*. The term may be misleading, however, suggesting that you're merely tacking a different border around the same old picture. Far from it. Reframing goes way beyond changing the context in which an idea lies. It means transforming the very idea itself. Reframing is not like redecorating; it's like gutting a house to its very foundation and rebuilding it to make it solid enough to last a lifetime.

How do I reframe what I'm thinking?

Reframing is a twofold, simple, and, yes, relatively easy process. It shouldn't take you long to get the hang of it. The first step is to identify your irrational, unhealthy beliefs, and the second is to rework them into rational, healthy ones. In the previous chapter you hopefully identified a slew of beliefs toxic to your becoming a "normal" eater, both from my list of irrational beliefs and from trolling your psyche to discover your rock-bottom thoughts about food, eating, weight, and your body. Each of these irrational beliefs can be transformed or reframed into one or more rational beliefs.

Let's take one from each of the four categories of irrational beliefs listed previously—food, eating, weight, and body—and you'll see how the process works. I'll use both general and "I" statements and give you a few rational beliefs for each irrational belief.

Food

Irrational Belief	Rational Beliefs
There are lots of bad and forbidden foods I shouldn't eat.	• There is no such thing as a bad or forbidden food. • Foods can be nutritious or not, but they don't have good or bad qualities. • No one can tell me what foods I should or shouldn't eat.

Eating

Irrational Belief	Rational Beliefs
It's shameful to eat too much.	• I refuse to be ashamed of myself no matter how much or how little I eat. • I accept myself even when I overeat. • "Normal" eaters occasionally eat too much.

Weight

Irrational Belief	Rational Beliefs
People who are more than 50 pounds overweight are disgusting.	• No one is disgusting because they have a large body. • I refuse to judge people by their weight. • Disgust should be reserved for people who do something genuinely hurtful or harmful to others.

Body

Irrational Belief	Rational Beliefs
I only deserve to be happy with myself when I'm thin.	• I can choose to be happy with myself whenever I want. • I deserve happiness at any weight. • Happiness is based on much more important things than a person's body size.

I hope you're getting the gist of what you have to do to make irrational beliefs rational. If you aren't sure if one of your beliefs is irrational, return to Chapter 3 and review Maultsby's assessment criteria. Remember, rational beliefs align with your life goals and enhance your life, so if one of your goals is to become a "normal" eater, your beliefs need to be compatible with "normal" eating. The more you practice turning irrational beliefs into rational ones, the easier the process will get.

What do "normal" eaters believe?

The funny thing about this question is that if you were to ask a "normal" eater what she believes about food and eating, she'd probably look at you with a blank stare and answer, "Gee, I'll have to think about that." Why would "normal" eaters pay any more attention to their beliefs than you previously did? They just munch merrily along through their daily food encounters without thinking much about why they're doing what they're doing.

A word of caution about idealizing "normal" eaters and imagining they're perfect human beings: eating "normally" doesn't necessarily mean that someone doesn't have problems dealing with their feelings or that they're free of other addictions, compulsions, obsessions, fears, health problems, or mental health concerns. They simply have their head on straight when it comes to food (and they do what comes naturally). They don't think much about what they believe because their attitudes and behaviors concerning food work for them in a healthy way. The reason you're exploring your beliefs is that your current behaviors and attitudes toward food make you miserable.

Using the categories and beliefs we set up previously, let's (yes, finally) examine the beliefs of "normal" eaters. A word about the four categories of beliefs. Generally, people who have disordered eating also have disordered thinking about their weight and bodies—generally, but not always. So the first two categories of beliefs, those about food and eating, reflect what "normal" eaters generally think.

But because it's hard for even "normal" eaters to escape societal, cultural, and family pressures about the shape and size of their bodies, the second two categories—weight and body—include healthy versus unhealthy beliefs that may or may not be held by "normal" eaters.

1. Reframing Beliefs About Food

- There are good foods (that is, low-calorie, low-fat) and bad foods (that is, high-calorie, high-fat).
  Food does not possess qualities such as good and bad, but it can be healthy or unhealthy for you.

- Food is the enemy.
  Food is neither friend nor foe.

- Food is dangerous and scary.
  Food is only dangerous and scary if it makes you sick.

- Food is scarce.
  Food is abundant.

- Food will make me fat.
  Tuning out my body's signals of hunger and fullness/ satisfaction will make me fat.

- Food takes care of me.
  Food takes care of my hunger; people take care of me. I take care of me.

- Food is love and comfort.
  Food is fuel and, often, pleasure.

- I need to be in tight control around food.
  I can be comfortable with food without being in tight control.

- Food should never, ever, under penalty of death—or worse—be wasted.
  If I've had enough to eat, more food inside me is a waste.

- I can never get enough food.
  I know when I've had enough food and feel pleasantly satisfied.

- I should eat only foods that are nutritious.
  It's fine to eat foods that are empty of nutrients if that's what my body craves and if I balance them out by eating healthy foods most of the time.

- I'll never learn to be satisfied with food.
  I'm learning and practicing being satisfied with food.

- I should never eat fattening foods.
  I can eat and enjoy high-calorie foods occasionally.

- Food will solve all my problems.
  Food can only solve the problem of hunger or craving.

- Eating low-cal food has to rule my life or I'll be as big as a horse.
  I trust my body to feed me in such a way that I remain at a natural, comfortable weight.

- If food is on my plate, I have to finish it.
  I can leave food on my plate, save it, or throw it away.

- Food is my best friend.
  My best friend is a person, and I don't expect food to give me what he or she can.

- Food is a good reward.
  There are many good rewards other than food.

- Food is my life.
  There is much more to my life than food.

2. Reframing Beliefs About Eating

- I have to eat fast before someone else gets more than I do.
  Eating is not competitive, and there's plenty of food for me.

- Eating will make me fat.
  I can enjoy food without worrying about putting on weight.

- If I don't think about what I'm eating, food can't hurt me or put pounds on me.
  Food can only hurt me if I eat past being full or satisfied.

- Eating is a painful process I wish I could do without.
  Eating is a pleasure, and I usually enjoy it.

- It's better to not eat and be thin than to be fat.
  Refusing to eat or eat enough is an unhealthy way to get and stay thin.

- I can't think about eating without becoming anxious.
  Thinking about eating makes me anticipate enjoyment.

- If I start eating something I like, I'll never stop.
  I can stop eating when I'm full or satisfied.

- Eating is better than feeling emotional pain or discomfort.
  Eating is an ineffective way to deal with emotional pain or discomfort.

- I can't stand eating around other people.
  I'm comfortable eating alone or with other people.

- Overeating is always a bad thing, and "normal" eaters never overeat.
  It's OK to overeat sometimes because everyone does.

- I'm ashamed of how I eat.
  I can eat without feeling ashamed.

- I never know what to eat.
  I generally know what I want to eat.

- I should always know what I want to eat.
  It's okay that I don't always know exactly what I want to eat.

- Hunger is scary.
  Hunger brings the anticipation of pleasure and satisfaction.

- I can't let myself feel hungry.
  My hunger just comes and goes on its own without permission.

- I should eat what other people want me to eat or what others are eating.
  Only I can decide what I want to eat.

- If I get together with people, eating has to be involved.
  If I get together with people, I don't care if we eat or not.

- My eating behaviors are so shameful, I can't let anyone see them.
  I'm not ashamed of any of my eating habits.

- Eating fills the emptiness inside me.
  The emptiness inside me is emotional and can't be filled by food. I can fill it up in other ways.

- Eating is the only pleasure I have in life.
  There are many things in life that bring me pleasure.

- Feeling good or bad about myself depends on what I eat or don't eat.
  How I feel about myself has nothing to do with what I eat or don't eat.

- Denying myself food shows I'm in control of my eating and, therefore, deprivation and restriction equal emotional strength.
  Strength and control come from exercising my personal power in the world, not from refusing to eat.

- If I can't find exactly what I want to eat, I feel deprived.
  I can feel fine even if I can't find exactly what I want to eat.

3. Reframing Beliefs About Weight

- I have to be thin.
  I don't have to be any particular weight or size.

- Thin equals a happy, successful, perfect life.
  People can be happy and successful at any size, but no one has a perfect life.

- I won't be happy or happy with myself until I lose weight.
  My happiness depends on who I am and what I do.

- Fat equals miserable, unhappy, and not deserving of or enjoying a good life.
  I deserve to be happy and to enjoy life at any weight.

- I should weigh myself every day.
  Weighing myself every day is unhealthy.

- I should never weigh myself.
  Weighing myself is unnecessary.

- If I didn't weigh myself, I wouldn't know what to eat.
  I know what to eat no matter what I weigh.

- Because people only see my fat body, I don't need to bother about my appearance.
  I enjoy making a good appearance.

- Being fat gets in the way of all the good things I want in life.
  I can enjoy life at any weight or size.

- Thin is more lovable than fat.
  I am lovable at whatever weight or size I am.

- I should weigh what the magazines and weight charts say I should.
  Eating "normally" is more important than what I weigh.

- Thin people are lucky and can eat whatever they want.
  Everyone has to make conscious choices about eating for their health.

- Large people should only eat low-calorie, low-fat foods.
  Large people need to eat a variety of foods, just like everyone else.

- The only way for me to be happy is to be or stay thin.
  I can be happy at any weight because happiness doesn't depend on body size.

- I'm too fat.
  I refuse to judge my body.

- Looking good is more important than being happy inside myself.
  Being happy with myself is more important than looking good.

- A person can never be too thin.
  People can be dangerously thin and die from it.

- Feeling proud or ashamed of myself depends on what I weigh.
  My feelings of pride or shame come from what I do, not what I weigh.

- No accomplishment of mine is as valuable as being or becoming a thin person.
  I have many accomplishments not related to my weight or body size.

- It's too scary to gain weight, even a pound.
  There's nothing scary about gaining weight.

- If I gain a pound or two, who knows when I'll stop gaining weight?
  It's OK if I gain a pound or two.

4. Reframing Beliefs About My Body

- I'll never be happy with my body.
  I'm going to start being happy with my body today.

- My body should be perfect.
  I accept my body as it is because there is no such thing as a perfect body.

- I can't trust my body to give itself the good care it needs.
  I trust my body to know what it needs in the way of good self-care.

- I can't trust my body to feed itself in a way that keeps me healthy and satisfied.
  I trust my body to make healthy food choices and to know when it's satisfied with food.

- My body is something to be ashamed of.
  I'm proud of my body.

- I can't love myself while I'm fat.
  I can love myself whether I'm fat or thin or in-between.

- I can only love myself while I'm thin.
  I can love myself whether I'm fat or thin or in-between.

- The purpose of a body is to look good.
  Bodies are meant to function, and my body is very functional.

- I'll never be proud of my body.
  I am proud of my body.

- The only thing about myself that I am proud of is my body.
  I am proud of many things about myself.

- I'm not in control of my body.
  My goal is to be comfortable in my body.

- If I can focus on controlling my body, I can avoid the fact that the rest of my life is a mess.
  By focusing exclusively on controlling my body, I'm missing a chance to deal with other areas of my life that need attention.

- My body will never learn when to say yes and no to food at the right times and in the right amounts.
  I can teach my body how to say yes and no to food at the right times and in the right amounts.

- What people think about my body is more important than what I think about it.
  What I think about my body is more important than what other people think of it.

- No one will ever love me if I'm fat.
  I'm lovable at any weight or body size.

So many irrational beliefs are caught up in the web of disordered eating that this list could go on and on. It is by no means exhaustive. You could tweak every irrational belief above and reframe it into a slightly different rational belief; some irrational beliefs are so complex that they can spawn two, three, or four rational ones. My point is to illustrate the chasm that lies between healthy and unhealthy thinking when it comes to food, eating, weight, and one's body.

"Normal" eating is about listening to your body and making healthy decisions. It's about pleasure, satisfaction, abundance, self-trust, good self-care, internal messages, and, most of all, *enjoying food*. Disordered eating—whether compulsive/emotional or restrictive—is about fear, deprivation, rigidity, childish gratification, mistrusting oneself, poor self-care, external messages, self-denial, and scary feelings. What is most striking about the comparison is that disordered thinking about eating has so little to do with actual put-it-on-your-plate-and-enjoy-it food!

Is it enough to change my beliefs about food, eating, weight, and my body?

No. Identifying food- and body-related beliefs is essential to becoming a "normal" eater, but stopping there is doing only part of the job. It's like straightening up one corner of your room and ignoring the rest: the mess continues to exist as a threat to your tidy little haven and may even eventually overrun it!

The goal is for *all* your beliefs to be healthy and rational. You want to be living from a functional set of what are called *core beliefs* so that all the beliefs that grow out of them will be affirming, positive, effective, and life-enhancing. Your core beliefs are your most basic assumptions about yourself and the world, your take on life; they contain your bedrock values and most firmly held convictions about how things should work. Think of them as the director concealed behind your mental curtain, orchestrating every mood and action of the play called *This Is Your Life*.

Your core beliefs—often unconsciously—have a hand in nearly everything you say and do. Therefore, along with identifying your specific healthy and unhealthy beliefs about food, eating, weight, and your body, you must also discover what your more general core beliefs are so that you know they are sound, functional, rational, and appropriate. Remember, becoming a "normal" eater goes beyond your relationship with food.

For example, if you believe that you don't deserve much in life, you're likely to trash yourself by constantly overeating junk food that makes you sick in body and spirit. If you believe you can't depend on other people to take care of you, you may turn to food rather than calling a friend. If you believe that you must keep others happy in order to receive love and affection, there's a good chance you'll make unsatisfying food choices rather than ruffle any feathers. If you believe that there's never enough of the good things in life, you'll likely be driven to inhale all the food on your plate. If you believe that your body isn't very valuable, you'll probably have little interest in nourishing it well.

Or, if you believe that feeling pleasure is wrong, you might say no to all the foods that taste good. If you believe there's nothing more important than appearance, you may strive for thinness at any price and forget about whether thin is healthy. If you believe that you can't trust your body to regulate its needs and wants, you may end up not responding to your hunger cues in fear of being unable to stop eating. If you believe that you don't have much inside to offer the world, you might think that a thin body will make you popular.

If you're feeling overwhelmed by the idea of examining your entire belief system —because, really, the only reason you picked up this book was to develop a friendlier relationship with food, not rehab your entire life—relax. It would be nearly impossible to explore your beliefs about food, eating, weight, and body in depth without bumping into some of your core beliefs along the way. The trick is to recognize them as core beliefs and carefully observe how they permeate (and often sabotage) your health and happiness. Once you've identified them, you can decide whether or not you need a major shopping excursion to the Belief Store to make some seriously needed exchanges.

You may still be unconvinced that unearthing your core beliefs will help you become a "normal" eater. Such an extensive excavation may seem like a huge effort and a waste of time merely to fix your relationship with food. "I just want to change my dysfunctional beliefs about food, weight, eating, and my body," you may be insisting. "Isn't that enough?"

Unfortunately, no. I think you'll realize fairly soon (and, perhaps, even be astounded) that your food- and body-related beliefs are highly reflective of how you think in major aspects of your life, and that revamping your core beliefs will move your whole cognitive system into healthy alignment by weeding out *all* the irrational beliefs that keep you in unhealthy relationship to yourself and others. Why go to the dentist to have a rotten tooth extracted but leave the diseased root? Better to remove the tooth and root at the same time.

How do I identify my core beliefs?

Learning how to identify your core beliefs is simple and—for once—fairly easy. The more aware you are of what you think and feel and the sharper your self-reflective powers, the easier it will be. You can probably identify about a dozen or so strongly held but not necessarily core beliefs right off the top of your head. Do you believe in God? Love at first sight? The value of education? That good should be rewarded and evil punished? That you're a sexy dancer? That money can buy happiness? That all politicians are cheats and liars? That your big nose prevents you from being attractive? That people are intrinsically selfish? That life is a bitch or a bowl of cherries? That you're a failure or a success? That because you came from a dysfunctional family, you'll never be happy?

Not all the above represent *core beliefs*. Remember, core beliefs are your most basic assumptions and expectations about yourself, life, and the world. They express your deepest values—the essence of who you are and what makes you tick.

If you're stumped and can't figure out how to identify your core beliefs, try browsing through a book of proverbs and deciding which are true—for you. Do you believe that absence makes the heart grow fonder? That practice makes perfect? That no man (or woman) is an island? That into every life a little rain must fall? That every cloud has a silver lining? That we reap what we sow? That all's well that ends well? That the apple doesn't fall far from the tree? That misery loves company? That the glass is half full or half empty?

What do I do when I've identified a set of core beliefs?

Once you've identified at least a dozen core beliefs, the next step is to put each one to Maultsby's test of whether or not it's rational. If the belief passes, great, keep and treasure it. If not, reframe it using the criteria you learned for reframing irrational eating-related beliefs. Whether the beliefs are specific to eating or they are core cognitions, the reframing process is the same.

If you need a few more incentives to begin examining and reframing your core beliefs, here they are. Having healthy, rational beliefs about yourself and the world will dramatically improve the quality of your life. If you've done a thorough job of rooting out dysfunctional core beliefs and replacing them with functional ones, your feelings will become more manageable, positive, and life-affirming. Emotionally, you'll feel more centered and comfortable in your own skin. Your attitudes about yourself and the world will be healthier, and you'll behave accordingly. As your behaviors change, you'll find yourself doing things that you never dreamed possible, taking new risks, acting in ways that would have been alien to your old core belief system. And your changed behaviors will reshape your feelings about yourself and support your new, healthy beliefs.

Here are some possible changes that might take place. Your expectations about yourself and others may become more realistic as your perfectionistic, all-or-nothing judgments gradually diminish. Your self-care may improve as you put yourself first and become more adept at saying yes and no in healthy balance. You may feel more sated and satisfied and know better when enough is really enough in myriad aspects of your life. You may develop more compassion for and trust in yourself and even learn to laugh at your foibles and mistakes. Being easier on yourself, you may become less critical of others. Shame and guilt may lessen to nontoxic, appropriate levels. You may feel more empowered, less of a victim of an unfair life. Relationships may change as you gravitate toward new, healthier friends and let go of relationships that make you unhappy and don't meet your emotional needs. You may feel surges of creativity and a desire to change your job or career. You may be less depressed and anxious, more hopeful and upbeat.

Moreover, having a sound set of core beliefs will make it infinitely easier for you to become a "normal" eater. If your brand-new, shiny belief says it's OK to ask for and expect comfort when you're upset, you'll be less likely to depend on General Mills or

Kraft or Häagen-Dazs® to do the job. If your new belief is that you can set your own goals for success, then you won't need to depend on our culture's twisted standard of ultra-thinness to feel good about yourself. If you've traded in your core belief that there's not enough of the good things in life for one that says that life is a banquet of rich possibilities, you won't feel driven to finish all the food on your plate. If you believe that you're a valuable, worthwhile person no matter what your parents told you, you'll eat only in ways that honor that highly esteemed self. If you've chosen to believe that it's nowhere near selfish to nurture and take care of yourself, you might begin by feeding your body the food it craves and needs.

A note of caution: revolutionizing your belief system can be scary. To reassure yourself that the process will not happen overnight, remember what you learned about change: that it is incremental and slow. Beginning a quest to transform your beliefs from dysfunctional to functional doesn't mean that you'll awaken one morning a different person with a fresh set of unfamiliar beliefs. Real life is not science fiction. We are not doing personality transplants here. You'll change only when you're ready, and you and you alone are in charge of the process. If you feel that you're taking too many risks or feeling emotionally alienated from yourself, gently put on the brakes. Regulate the pace to make it comfortable for you, neither warp speed nor slow as a slug.

You may be surprised by changes that seem to come out of the blue (*I said that? Boy, that's so unlike me! I can't believe what I just did!*). Other people may notice that you seem different before you do. They may approve or disapprove, but you're the only one who can decide how and who you want to be. You may experience a few shocks to the system, but for the most part, change will be gradual and evenly paced, just as it should be. My guess is that, if anything, change will come too slowly for you, not too quickly.

The bottom line is that becoming a "normal" eater will affect more than your relationship with food. It will impact every inch of your life, every minute of your existence, all for the better. So take the challenge of revamping your core beliefs, and prepare yourself for a happier, healthier life.

How do I connect my core beliefs to my thinking about food, eating, weight, and my body?

Amazingly, even if you were to change only your core beliefs and not your specific food, eating, weight, and body beliefs, you would still notice a surprising shift in the quality of your life. Believing that it's possible—and even preferable—to trust yourself and other people, that it's a relief to depend on and get help from others, that the world is made up of shades of gray rather than only black and white, that you have power to change your life for the better, and that you're a valuable, unique person cannot help but improve your relationship with food and your own body. Once your core beliefs are healthier and more functional, you might even find that your beliefs about eating and weight fall right into line behind them without too much added work.

However, if you want to work specifically to tie your food and body beliefs into your core beliefs, here's a process that I think you'll find surprisingly easy. It consists of three basic steps: 1) Identify the eating- or body-related behavior you want to change; 2) Identify the irrational eating- or body-related belief underlying the behavior; and 3) Identify the irrational core belief that underlies the food/weight/body-related belief. Here are some examples.

Example A

1) Identify the eating/body behavior you want to change.

Behavior: Finishing all the food on my plate.

2) Identify the irrational eating/body belief underlying the behavior.

Belief: I am being wasteful if I don't finish all the food on my plate.

3) Identify the irrational core body belief underlying the behavior.

Core Belief: Being wasteful is an unforgivable sin.

Example B

1) Identify the eating/body behavior you want to change.

Behavior: Denying myself food when I am hungry.

2) Identify the irrational eating/body belief underlying the behavior.

Belief: If I start eating I won't be able to stop.

3) Identify the irrational core body belief underlying the behavior.

Core Belief: I need to maintain strict control over my body.

Example C

1) Identify the eating/body behavior you want to change.

Behavior: Weighing myself every day.

2) Identify the irrational eating/body belief underlying the behavior.

Belief: I need to weigh myself to know what I should or shouldn't eat.

3) Identify the irrational core body belief underlying the behavior.

Core Belief: I can't trust my body to know what it needs.

Of course, you could probably come up with a variety of eating beliefs and core beliefs that underlie each behavior. For example, regarding finishing the food on your plate, another belief might be *I will be punished or humiliated if I waste food,* and the core belief might be *People deserve punishment or humiliation for being wasteful.* Or, the belief might be *If I don't finish my food, people will think I'm not grateful for it,* and the core belief might be *I must always feel grateful for what I am given.*

Technically, there's no limit to how many core beliefs you can identify. Just remember, core beliefs reflect your most basic assumptions about yourself and the world. You want enough variety to cover all the important aspects of your life, but not so many that there's duplication or too much specificity. Conversely, when you're identifying eating- and body-related beliefs, the more the merrier. Here's where you want to be specific, so that you know exactly what you believe about food, eating, weight, and your body. Here are a couple of ways to start uncovering the core beliefs that underlie your food problems.

You can begin by looking for core beliefs in the following areas: work/play, love, parents, emotions, happiness/unhappiness, family, success/failure, learning, trust, reward/punishment, dependence/independence, relationships, community, children, goals, support, authority, self. Notice the particular core beliefs that may fuel your disordered eating and drive you to be critical of your weight and unaccepting of your body. Or start with food, eating, weight, and body-related words such as abundance/deprivation, restriction, excess, enough, fat, thin, large, tiny, entitlement, fullness, satisfied, hunger, scale, clothes, appearance, visible/invisible, acceptable/unacceptable, lovable/despicable, empty, denial, substantial/insubstantial, starving, unfulfilled, feeding.

It may take a while to get the hang of identifying your beliefs. *Remember, there are no right or wrong answers.* However, there is a felt sense of accuracy or a resonance when you're right on the money—a ping of recognition, an internal "Gee whiz, that's it!" The more extensively you work on your beliefs, the easier it will be to sift through them and choose just the right match or matches for each behavior or feeling you want to change.

No matter where you begin the process of identifying core beliefs, you'll end up in the same place: enjoying a better life!

6

FEELINGS AND FEEDING

*Can't I Pay Someone to Do This
Feeling Stuff for Me?*

Nowhere is the gulf between "normal" and dysfunctional eaters more evident than in the way they handle feelings. For "normal" eaters, feelings and food operate in two separate orbits that only occasionally, if ever, intersect. Sure, "normal" eaters sometimes temporarily disconnect from their bodies and eat compulsively—it's the bottom of the ninth, bases are loaded, the Sox are down by one, and the eater is elbow-deep in a bag of Fritos®. But "normal" eaters feel no magical connection between feeling and food, and they are as likely to *lose* their appetite during surges of emotion as they are to eat. For "normal" eaters, *feeding is feeding* and *feeling is feeling*.

But for disordered eaters, food and feeling have a special, unique relationship. You use eating—or not eating—and weight worries as a way to manage uncomfortable feelings that you may not even realize exist. If you're a compulsive/emotional eater, feeling and feeding are interwoven like fibers in a fabric; your heart and mouth are no longer separate organs. *I feel* and *I eat* become IFEELIEAT. If you're a restrictive eater, rigid efforts to control your weight and body and *not* eat distract you from experiencing painful emotions and affirm that everything is OK.

Either way, the goal is the same: to avoid feeling uncomfortable at any cost. Smother your feelings in food, funnel your emotional energy into shopping and cooking, mold your body into a machine that needs nothing (neither food nor feelings), obsess over eating and weight so you won't think about the messes in your life. Feelings need not even be intense or overwhelming to trigger your desire to run from them; the tiniest flicker of unease can set off a chain reaction.

As an emotional/compulsive eater, food is your emergency rescue squad, rushing in to save you from emotional distress—disappointment, frustration, confusion, loneliness, helplessness. "Everything's under control," it assures you. "Relax, we'll take it from here." And there food stays, with its soothing bedside manner and false assurances, keeping you anesthetized until the pain is sucked dry, bitten to pieces, swallowed whole, chewed to a pulp, ground down to nothing, chomped to death.

As a restrictive eater, your excessive and obsessive control over what you can and can't eat and what you should weigh—counting calories, limiting portion sizes, labeling foods good and bad, worrying about what you ate or might eat—is a misguided attempt to manage your emotional landscape. Because upsetting emotions cause you to feel out of control (They do that to all of us!), you focus instead on something within your power. Your preoccupation with eating as little as possible and staying thin replaces authentic upset and natural feelings. Most important, because depriving yourself of food and being ultraslim are sanctioned and even extolled in our culture (as opposed to being fat, which is almost universally scorned), you have no idea that you're missing the point with food *and* feeling.

But life being what it is, you have to stop eating or obsessing about food *sometime*—to take care of the kids, go to work or school, shop, clean, call Mom, shower, wash the car, go to the bank or the bathroom, sleep, keep appointments. And when you stop, back come the feelings: they didn't disappear after all. You're disappointed, saddened, scared—but, of course, you knew they'd return because they always do.

The problem is that there's a big part of you that really doesn't want to know that food as your healer is a sham, an artful con, a dumb ruse; that the joke, unfortunately, is on you. That's why you continue to eat and obsess about food: to postpone that inevitable headlong slam into the wall of reality, mouth wide open, or tightly shut, when the pain comes rushing back.

You may be grumbling to yourself, OK, I give, fixation on food isn't the answer to uncomfortable feelings. So what is? I'll answer that question in a little while. But, as they say in AA, first things first. To know what to do with feelings, you need to understand their purpose. The simple answer is that just as food is meant to be eaten, feelings are meant to be felt! Here's why.

What's the purpose of feelings?

This excellent question cuts right to the heart of the issue. Think of your feelings as guides to your internal world, much as your senses—touch, smell, sight, taste, hearing—help you navigate the external world. Someone yells, "Fire!" or you smell smoke, and an instant later you're racing out the door. When you hear chalk screech across a board, you automatically jerk your head away from the sound. You tilt your head in the direction of a memorable melody. When the bathwater is too hot, you yank out your foot before it scalds, but when the water is just right, you sink slowly into it, close your eyes, and let out a sigh of heavenly satisfaction.

Once you understand the function of your senses, you'll find it easier to understand the function of your feelings. Senses steer you clear of danger and threat and guide you toward experiences that will enhance your life. That's their purpose. You automatically retreat from the growl of a bear and advance toward the purr of a kitten. The most basic purpose of your senses is to keep you out of harm's way, alive and enjoying life. Biologically speaking, senses help you thrive, ensuring that you stick around and enjoy the show—and perhaps even take some time to propagate the species.

Put another way, your senses direct you toward pleasure in life and away from pain. Freud was right on the money with his idea of the *pleasure principle*. Today's neurobiologists are able to use high-tech brain imaging to study the pleasure and reward centers in the brain as well as the neurotransmitters, or chemical messengers, that both enhance pleasure and diminish pain.

Both senses and emotions connect you to the world outside yourself, only senses do it in a more blatant way. A continuous cramp in the arch of your foot has you limping to a podiatrist, but where does a pain in your heart take you? To the refrigerator? To the scale? I can't say it often enough. Your feelings, as well as your senses, are meant to direct you away from ultimate pain and move you toward ultimate pleasure. That's it, their basic function. Uncomfortable feelings are not there to plague you, drive you crazy, make you depressed or sick, or cause you stress. Feelings, like food, have no hidden motives. All feelings are meant to do is provide the information you vitally need to make your life better and keep you from emotional and physical harm.

So you see, in order for emotions to help you stay alive and thrive, you have to experience them, in much the same way as you experience your senses! If you were unable to taste, smell, see, feel, or hear, you'd be in a real pickle. If you turned off your senses, you'd never see the train rushing at you, or hear the sharp squeal of its brakes.

Without our senses, how would we be able to tell what was life-threatening from what was life-enhancing? We couldn't—game over! My guess is that the very thought of losing any one of your senses strikes terror in your heart, that you value each and every sense with a reverence and possessiveness you may not even realize until you contemplate losing it. Without your senses, you wouldn't be able to distinguish a pea from a pebble, embers from ashes, friend from foe, or the bellow of a French horn from the blast of a 10-ton truck.

Are all feelings created equal?

All of your feelings are equally important in transmitting information to you—their primary purpose. Think of them as your private couriers bringing you special deliveries, your very own headline news service, except that the bulletins flash not every hour, but every second of your waking life (and, through dreams, your sleeping life). The raw (pun intended) data that emotions carry—fierce disappointment at a friend's betrayal or heart-pounding dread when you're called into your boss's office—is every bit as valuable as what you learn from your senses—that the sun is too hot, the water too cold. But if you continue to shoot the messenger, how will you ever get the message?

If you keep the volume of your emotions turned down low, how will you make out what they're saying? If you're not listening attentively, you may hear only half the message, get only the barest gist of it, or fail to pick up its shades of meaning. You may selectively tune in to only the emotional stations you like best (joy, contentment, confidence, competence, feeling loved and valued) and tune out the unpleasant. Paying attention to every single station on your emotional receiver may feel too hard, too time consuming, too unfamiliar, too depressing, too scary. So you give up and stop listening—and start eating or worrying about your weight.

If a bicycle ran over your foot, you'd probably be in pain and would get rapid medical attention. But if a lover runs over your heart, what do you do? You feel that pinch of pain and head for the linguini or decide you'll skip lunch because maybe he'll come back if you're thinner. You might as well run an IV of novocaine straight to your heart and be done with feeling forever.

The problem is that by avoiding emotional pain, you avoid the wisdom and warnings embedded in it—do this and don't do that. Troubling emotions often signal just that—trouble. And if you miss the signal, you're likely to get hurt down the line. If you've gotten this far in life, you're probably in the habit of paying attention to the whistle at railroad crossings. But if you stop listening, you might be hit by a train before you finish this book! A similar death sentence—emotional if not physical—awaits you if you continue to ignore the signals from your heart.

Why do I avoid uncomfortable emotions?

The simple answer is because you're human. Remember Freud's theory that we move toward pleasure and away from pain? On one level, that's all you're doing. You're in good company; the rest of the human race is trying to do the same thing. *The first reason you have difficulty staying with distressing feelings is that you're hardwired to move toward pleasure and away from pain.*

To give a more complete answer for why you turn away from troubling emotions, we will return to the theory of cognitive-behavioral therapy. *The second reason it's hard to experience the entire spectrum of your emotions is that you may have irrational beliefs about feelings, which discourage you from experiencing them.* These beliefs act as gatekeepers of your emotions, giving a stamp of approval to some (it's OK to feel elation) and turning away others (it's not OK to feel helpless).

Here are a number of irrational beliefs that may prevent you from experiencing difficult emotions.

- I should never have to experience emotional pain.
- I don't like feeling bad, so I shouldn't have to.
- I should always strive to be happy.
- Emotional pain has no point or function.
- Painful emotions will either drive me crazy or kill me.
- Once I feel the feeling, I will be stuck in it forever.
- Emotional pain will knock me down and I'll never get up.
- To make a good impression, I should always keep a smile on my face.
- If I'm not pleasant and upbeat, other people will be upset with me.

- It's weak to give in to uncomfortable feelings.
- Strong people don't have negative or painful feelings.
- If I always do the right thing, I can avoid unpleasant feelings.
- It's better to just ignore bad feelings so they'll go away.
- I am my feelings; that is, if I *feel* bad, I *am* bad.
- I shouldn't dwell on my feelings because I can't do anything about them.
- It's self-indulgent to keep thinking about how I feel.
- If I allow myself to feel negative feelings, I'll behave badly.
- I shouldn't worry about what I'm feeling, only about what I'm doing.

Every one of the above beliefs is irrational and unhealthy, but I bet that you recognize at least some of them as near and dear to your heart. These beliefs are why you have difficulty staying connected to painful feelings. Remember, change the belief, and the feeling falls in line behind it. It can be difficult at first to decide what it means to have healthy, rational beliefs about emotions and to construct a wholly healthy cognitive system. So to make things easier for you, I've turned the irrational beliefs above into rational ones.

Irrational Belief	Rational Beliefs
I should never have to feel pain.	• Everyone experiences emotional pain sometime in their life. • Emotional pain is valuable because it gives me information about myself and my world. • It's normal to feel emotional pain.

I don't like feeling bad, so I shouldn't have to.	• Just because I don't enjoy feeling bad doesn't mean I should cut off my feelings. • I do lots of things I don't like because I know they will improve my life. • I'll feel worse in the long run if I don't feel my feelings.
I should always strive to be happy.	• Being happy all the time is neither possible nor genuine. • Feeling unhappy is as natural as feeling happy. • Nothing bad will happen to me if I'm not happy.
Emotional pain has no point or function.	• Emotional pain is a warning that something isn't right and I'm hurting. • The point of emotional pain is to keep me emotionally safe. • Emotional pain has an ultamite life-enhancing function.
Painful emotions will either drive me crazy or kill me.	• I can bear painful emotions through my own resources or with the help of other people • Bearing painful emotions will neither drive me crazy nor kill me. • Painful emotions feel dangerous and harmful, but they aren't.

Once I feel the feeling I will be stuck in it forever.	• Feelings come and go. • Feelings change over time. • I know how to feel my feelings and let them go.
Emotional pain will knock me down and I'll never get up.	• I have the ability to withstand and learn from emotional pain. • I become a stronger person through managing my emotional pain. • I don't have to fear emotional pain.
To make a good impression, I'll always keep a smile on my face.	• Being real matters more than making a false impression. • A false impression is not a good impression—no one feels happy all the time. • I don't need to impress anyone but myself.
Other people will be upset with me for feeling unpleasant.	• It's OK if other people are upset that I have unpleasant feelings. • It's nobody's business what I feel or don't feel. • I'm entitled to have any feelings I want, pleasant or unpleasant.

It's weak to give in to uncomfortable feelings.	• Only people who fear their feelings think that it's weak to feel them. • Experiencing and tolerating uncomfortable feelings will make me stronger. • Experiencing feelings is not the same as giving in to them.
Strong people don't have negative or painful feelings.	• Everyone has negative or painful feelings. • There is no such thing as being strong all the time. • Emotional strength and resilience come only from learning to bear uncomfortable feelings.
If I always do the right thing, I can avoid unpleasant feelings.	• It's part of being human to have unpleasant feelings. • No matter how I live, I will have unpleasant feelings. • There's no right way to live, and I can't avoid making mistakes.
It's better to just ignore bad feelings so they'll go away.	• Bad feelings will always come back if I ignore their message. • I don't have to ignore my feelings because they'll go away on their own after I have taken in their message. • I don't have to push bad feelings away just to make myself more comfortable.

I am my feelings; that is, if I *feel* bad, I *am* bad.	• What I feel is separate from who I am. • There is no inevitable connection between feeling something and being something. • Good people sometimes feel bad.
I shouldn't dwell on my feelings because I can't do anything about them.	• I can change my feelings by changing my beliefs. • I can change my feelings by changing my behavior • By feeling my feelings, I receive their message.
It's self-indulgent to keep thinking about how I feel.	• To be emotionally healthy, I have to keep in touch with my feelings. • Thinking about how I feel is necessary and important to my well-being. • No one can tell me what I should or shouldn't do with my feelings.
If I allow myself to feel negative feelings, I'll behave badly.	• I can contain my feelings and not let them spill into my behavior. • Feeling negative feelings may prevent me from acting out negative behaviors. • Sometimes it's necessary to behave badly.

I shouldn't worry about what I'm feeling, only about what I'm doing.	• I have to know what I'm feeling to do what's in my best interest. • If I pay attention to what I'm feeling, what I'm doing will reflect my real needs. • I don't have to worry about what I'm feeling, I need only feel my feelings.

Notice that the negative connotation given to emotional pain in the irrational belief is changed to positive in each reframing, promoting a rational belief that is appropriate to emotions. Rational beliefs help you manage your emotions effectively and increase your power over your feelings and behavior. Whenever you're reframing beliefs about your feelings, remember that the new rational belief you create should uplift you and leave you feeling better about yourself. It's OK to feel scared or a bit uncertain about whether you can actually live by the belief. Try it on for size and wear it around for a while, as you would a new pair of shoes. The point is to make sure that the belief is life-enhancing, supported by evidence, and will further your life goals.

Another reason you avoid emotional discomfort is that you may not know what to do, once you recognize you're in pain. To illustrate, let's return to the analogy of the bicycle running over your foot. Unless you were in physical shock or excruciating pain (or had unhealthy beliefs about how you should react to physical pain!), it's likely that you'd fairly quickly come up with a workable plan of action. You'd cope, deal with the pain, and try to do what makes sense and is best for you. It's unlikely that you'd lie there for too long without wondering whether to go to the ER, phone someone, limp home, call out to a passerby, pop an analgesic or painkiller, or chase after the person on the bike. You might take a moment to decide what action to take, but then you'd make up your mind fairly quickly. If you were emotionally healthy, you'd register the throbbing in your foot as a signal that it needed medical attention, and you'd make that your first priority.

Optimum health means attending to both physical and emotional injury as quickly as possible. Not surprisingly, this can be difficult when the pain is not in your foot but in your heart. It may feel too awful to focus on your pain. If all you want to do is flee from distress, how can you take in pain's message or attend to healing it?

If someone runs over your heart and all you want to do is get rid of the pain, you might panic and fail to act in ways that are in your ultimate best interest. You might make choices that will diminish, eliminate, or postpone the pain, but won't keep you happy and healthy in the long run. You can't know what to *do* unless you first know what you *feel*; you can't fix something if you don't know what's wrong! Feeling provides a diagnosis for the problem. If all you want to do is stop the pain, you will never, ever heal an emotional problem.

How come I don't know how to deal with emotional pain effectively?

At this point, you might be wondering how you developed into a person who is unable to experience and cope with emotional pain without abusing food. The answer is that no one modeled or taught you how to handle your feelings effectively and appropriately. *Therefore, the reason you have difficulty in this area is that you lack effective skills in dealing with feelings.* You probably don't know how to parasail either, if you never watched anyone do it and no one ever showed you how.

Effective emotional management is a learned and learnable skill. It's not innate; it's something we have to be taught. If you didn't learn how to manage your emotions effectively in your childhood, here's your second chance. All it takes is awareness and practice. The more you do it, the easier it gets. If you don't eat or starve your way through a feeling or find any of the other gazillion seductive ways you have to distract yourself from what's going on inside you, you'll get the hang of it. Later in this chapter I'll tell you exactly what to do when you have the stirrings of an uncomfortable feeling.

As to how you became inept at handling feelings, let's simply say that if your role models didn't have a healthy attitude toward experiencing all their feelings, they couldn't teach you how to deal appropriately and effectively with yours. This includes not only negative ones—because if you believe you don't deserve joy, success, and happiness, these also can feel mighty icky and unfamiliar. If your parents or caretakers did any of the following on a regular basis, they lacked the skills necessary to deal with their own feelings (and yours!):

- Drank, drugged, binged on food or starved, purged, gambled, worked, shopped, or pursued any activity addictively
- Were abusive sexually, physically, emotionally, or verbally to you or others
- Regularly neglected or ignored your feelings
- Gave you or other family members the silent treatment or often withdrew emotionally

- Consistently placed you or your siblings in the position of inappropriately taking care of *their* emotional needs
- Pretended that they were fine and never unhappy
- Lived rigidly with excessive, unfair rules about most things in life
- Habitually acted out through dangerously risky behavior

All of the above behaviors isolate people from their emotions and are signs of mismanaged feelings. Your parents couldn't teach you what they didn't know how to do themselves. So here you are today, still unskilled in experiencing and dealing with your emotions and turning to or away from food for salvation.

If you could learn other life skills, you can learn how to handle your feelings. Skillfully managing your feelings will have a major impact on your relationship with food. It's the single most important—and probably the hardest—change you will have to make to become a "normal" eater. Moreover, it will teach you how to be so finely in tune with yourself that you will be able to find the authentic happiness and success you want and deserve in life.

If I'm hard-wired to avoid pain, how will I learn to manage uncomfortable feelings?

The best way to start exploring how to manage emotional pain is to back up and get an overview of the subject. After all, heartache has been around since the beginning of humankind, and there is no shortage of theory or opinion on the subject. The more you understand about emotions, the better you'll do at using them to your advantage and the less inclined you'll be to use your relationship with food to avoid them.

Consider, for example, that emotional dissonance and discomfort come in many flavors. There's the razor sharp slash to the heart that's over in an instant but nearly takes your breath away; and the dull, throbbing ache in your soul that never seems to leave you. There's the short-term pain that leads to long-term absence of pain, or even to pleasure, when you refuse a date with the same old cad who always breaks your heart. You may feel a pang of discomfort as you decline the date, and your discomfort may even stick around for awhile, but sooner or later you'll feel better knowing that you're preventing future pain and giving yourself a chance for love to bloom in more fertile soil.

British psychoanalyst R. D. Laing has an invaluable view of pain. He maintains that "There is a great deal of pain in life, and perhaps the only pain that can be avoided is the pain of trying to avoid pain." The thought is deep and complex, so you may need to read the quote a couple of times to really get it. It is one of my favorites, and sits prominently in my office for all to read (and to serve as a reminder to me, as well). Laing is telling us that we are helpless to escape pain, but that we *do* have the power to choose our poison. He's saying we'll feel pain now or later, in this way or that. There's no escaping it. When we stop trying to run from emotional pain, we can take control over it rather than letting it control us. Laing reinforces the conviction of cognitive-behavioral therapy that the only path to lessening discomfort is through informed, rational choice.

Buddhist teaching differentiates between two types of pain: involuntary and voluntary suffering. Involuntary suffering is an innate part of life, the price we pay for renting space on the planet, the result of being alive. We know we'll encounter loss and failure, unhappiness and sickness, grief and sorrow, because that's what it means to be human. Involuntary suffering is inescapable, and we cannot control it. People get sick and die or make mistakes that tragically affect our life. The clouds burst and rain on our parade. The thing to remember about involuntary suffering is that we need not go looking for it; it finds us.

Voluntary suffering, on the other hand, is generated by wanting—a house, a car, a new outfit, peace and quiet, to be a doctor, to live in the country, to be thin, to be a "normal" eater, to be healthy, to continue living, to be loved, to be free from pain. Pain is the dark night that exists between wanting and not having. Even wanting to *not* want is a kind of wanting. Because there's no way to avoid wanting, we are all destined to suffer voluntarily to some extent throughout our lives. However, we can decide what we want and, therefore, how much we will suffer.

According to Buddhism, one way to diminish suffering is by becoming aware of your wants and detaching from them. For example, you want to arrive at your favorite restaurant by seven o'clock to grab a table before the evening rush, but en route you get a flat. Your frustration, annoyance, impatience, helplessness—your suffering—is caused by *wanting* to get to the restaurant at a specific time. But if you tell yourself, "C'est la vie, I'll go another night" or, "I'll relax while I wait for a table," you're no longer plagued by wanting. You have become the instrument to end your suffering. Or, say you have been thinking that you hate your body and want desperately to be thinner, a terrible kind of self-imposed suffering. By deciding to accept your body at whatever weight you are and detaching from the desire for thinness, you can avoid suffering. You may even find yourself making healthier food choices.

You may be wondering if I'm recommending that you live life without desire. Of course not. Suffering voluntarily is often the only direct path to future gain, benefit, or pleasure. You get immunization shots; sit in traffic; wait in line at the movies; put yourself last for your children; take long, boring plane rides; sweat it out at the gym; pay your taxes; and work hard to save for retirement. There is a point to this suffering, and you choose to suffer because it has a life-enhancing payoff.

But if you are one of those people who suffer unnecessarily because you continually put yourself in harm's way, that's a different story. You might as well play chicken with a bus or go over Niagara Falls in a barrel. Here are some examples of voluntary suffering for no good end: going out with a jerk who's abusive and whom all your friends hate, weighing yourself every day and giving the scale the power to make or break your day, trying to be perfect, smoking cigarettes, waiting to be happy until you lose weight, staying in a crummy job you can't stand, enduring intense physical pain because you're afraid to go the doctor or hospital, refusing to feed yourself when you're starving, punishing your body with excessive exercise, denying your true wants because you're ashamed of them, always trying to be emotionally strong. In all these instances you're making the choice to suffer and your wounds are self-inflicted, but for no valid reason. If you don't want the pain, then put down the knife! You cannot completely avoid voluntary suffering—after all, everyone wants *something*—but you can minimize the pain you inflict on yourself by making constructive choices not to suffer unnecessarily or excessively. The point is to have healthy wants that can be effectively met and that will enhance your well-being.

Regarding food, involuntary suffering presupposes that there will be times when you won't get exactly what you want to eat—you're on the road, in a meeting, the kids are screaming, or the restaurant is closed or out of your favorite dish. Such is life. You register the loss and move on. Voluntary suffering is being so furious and disappointed that you can't get what you want that you eat two helpings of something you don't want and then feel sick as a dog, or you refuse to eat anything because you didn't get your first, perhaps "safer" food choice.

How do "normal" eaters manage their feelings?

Some manage their feelings well, and some don't. Although it's true that to become a "normal" eater, *you* have to learn how to manage your feelings more effectively, this doesn't mean that all "normal" eaters deal with their feelings in an appropriate way. They may have other bad habits or vices that help them avoid or minimize emotional distress. They may drink, use drugs, work, shop, exercise, clean, focus excessively on others, or gamble too much. They may isolate and withdraw from loved ones or take unnecessary, hazardous risks. They may set up rigid rules to live by, hold unrealistic expectations of themselves and others, and try to be perfect. They may become depressed, highly anxious, abusive, or even suicidal.

However, the one thing they do not do habitually is use food to help manage their feelings. Think about the "normal" eaters you know (if you know any). Do they have any bad habits or addictions? Do they model effective emotional management? Might you have a better handle on your highs and lows and what to do with feelings than they do? "Normal" eaters are not necessarily more skilled at handling feelings than you are, so be careful not to idealize them. Try to model your eating around the rules they *eat* by, not the rules they *live* by, unless you think they're supremely mentally healthy individuals.

Of course, "normal" eaters may occasionally turn to or away from food when they're upset, just as the nonalcoholic may pour herself a drink once in a while when stressed to the max, or some-one who is not a drug addict may take a sedative to get to sleep now and then, rather than toss and turn all night. The point is that, unlike disordered eaters, "normal" eaters do not depend on food—eating it, thinking about it, or depriving themselves of it—to manage their emotions.

What feelings are the most difficult to manage?

Although everyone has a different reaction to specific emo-tions, it's possible to offer some generalities about feelings. First of all, we humans enjoy a sense of comfort in grouping feelings into categories of "good" and "bad," and there's no question that the sunnier ones are preferable. "Good" feelings are ones that are pleasant and include:

joy	connection	elation
happiness	surprise	bliss
success	comfort	serenity
hope	satisfaction	contentment
love	pride	ecstasy
achievement	pleasure	freedom
excitement	delight	independence
affection	anticipation	worthiness

"Bad" feelings are ones that are unpleasant:

sadness	uncertainty	hurt
grief	humiliation	pain
disappointment	loneliness	panic
stress	despair	regret
helplessness	frustration	trapped
failure	distress	threatened
sorrow	disgust	anxiety
shame	anguish	worthlessness
guilt	embarrassment	hatred
fear	envy	terror
anger	jealousy	horror
bitterness	rejection	remorse
boredom	abandonment	emptiness
confusion	hopelessness	depression

Second, we naturally feel overwhelmed by "bad" feelings when they swoop down on us en masse. We handle them better when they behave and form a single line so that we can experience them one at a time. We love simplicity; we crave order. But, like wild creatures, feelings often travel in packs. *One at a time*, we insist, but they couldn't care less and keep coming. We are just getting over our disappointment at not being invited to a friend's party when rejection, dejection, jealousy, hurt, worthlessness, and helplessness come charging in and practically knock the wind out of us.

Third, we like to keep things simple. Not only do we prefer to experience only one feeling at a time, but we'd rather not mix our "good" and "bad" feelings. For example, let's say that a favorite colleague has landed a dream job in another state, and you're genuinely thrilled for her. While wishing her all the best, you notice you have other feelings about her move: sadness at the loss of a confidante, envy or shame because you feel trapped in the same old job while your colleague is on the fast track, fear that you'll be stuck with extra work until the boss hires someone new, anxiety about what kind of coworker will replace her.

Conflicting and polarized feelings can be difficult to hold on to simultaneously. So to feel more comfortable, you might deny or shuck off one set of feelings, usually the "negative" ones. You may feel thrilled for your colleague and deny your hurt feelings because you think you shouldn't have them or because they make you feel emotionally torn. However, good mental health dictates being able to tolerate opposing feelings and bear the tension of ambivalence. In fact, being able to hold two opposing feelings at the same time is a sign of emotional intelligence.

A fourth generality complicates our emotional landscape even further: we not only have feelings, but we have feelings *about* our feelings. This statement brings us back to how cognitions affect emotions. Returning to the example of not being invited to a friend's party, let's say you're feeling angry at her for excluding you. You think you've been a comrade extraordinaire, and you feel left out to the point of wanting to cry or scream. However, if you were brought up to feel that it's wrong to feel sorry for yourself, you might deny your hurt or anger. You might feel ashamed of these "selfish" feelings and tell yourself that it was just an oversight that you weren't invited and that you're a bad person to think critically of your friend. The shame is a secondary feeling, *a reaction to* the hurt and anger that were your primary feelings. It is based on the erroneous belief that it's wrong to feel certain things.

You might have a similar reaction to your colleague leaving work. If your belief is that you should feel only happy for someone else's success and ignore your other reactions, you might feel guilty or selfish that you're angry and sad and anxious about the loss. The guilt is a secondary feeling, a response to your primary feelings of anger, sadness, and anxiety. A problem arises when your irrational belief system dictates how you *should* feel about having these feelings and generates concurrent or subsequent feelings of guilt, shame, inadequacy, or helplessness.

Moreover, although you might think that you want to have only "good" feelings, they may actually make you uneasy. In fact, this uneasiness is such a common reaction to feeling good about yourself that you may not identify it as a source of your dysfunctional relationship with food! Why would you be uneasy about feeling pleasant feelings? Well, of course, because of what you believe about them. Are you using them to cover up or deny other "less acceptable" feelings? Do you believe you deserve to feel good? That happiness will last, or that someone or something will take it away? That it's OK for you to feel happy when others aren't? That it's wrong or sinful or selfish to feel good, and there will be a price to pay?

Naturally, if you have any of these assumptions or if feeling good is an unfamiliar state, you'll likely end up feeling bad about feeling good! And what better way to undo the positive feelings than by having a little nosh when you're not hungry or a big, big nosh that seems as if it could go on all night, until you run out of food? Or sabotaging your good feelings by punishing your body and making yourself suffer? This may take the form of depriving yourself of food when you're hungry or denying yourself the foods you really crave.

Emotional balance and wise management mean being equally tolerant of "good" and "bad" feelings. Of course, no one enjoys unpleasant feelings, just as no one finds pleasure in going to the dentist, the doctor, or the hospital. The fact that we dislike certain activities should not, necessarily, prevent us from doing them. Consciously or unconsciously, we understand that they fall under the category of involuntary suffering. As I've said before, pleasure and pain are part of life and must both be embraced in order to live fully and healthily—and to avoid having a dysfunctional relationship with food! Sometimes, "the way out is the way through."

OK, so what do I need to do to manage my feelings effectively?

If you're tuned in to cognitive-behavioral thinking, you already know the answer. Remember the maxim: Change the belief, change the feeling and the behavior. Transform your irrational, unhealthy beliefs about feelings—"good" and "bad," multiple, conflicting, primary and secondary—into rational, healthy beliefs, and you'll automatically manage your emotions more effectively. The more strongly anchored you are in your new belief system, the less likely you'll be to eat or restrict your food intake when you're emotionally distressed, and the greater the probability that you'll eat "normally."

You can use the reframed beliefs about having painful feelings listed earlier in this chapter to start reforming your cognitions. Here are some additional rational beliefs that will create a healthier climate for exploring, accepting, and handling your emotions.

- Because feelings are not facts, I can alter them by changing my beliefs.
- The nature of feelings is that they come and go.
- Feelings are informative, and knowing what I feel will enhance my life.
- No feeling is impossible to bear with the help of others and my own emotional resources.
- Turning to others for help with my feelings will prevent me from turning to eating or not eating to take care of emotional wounds.
- Learning to manage my emotions will take time, skill, practice, patience, and compassion for myself.
- Feelings are neither good nor bad; they just are.
- I accept all of my feelings without judging them.
- Whatever I feel has been felt (and managed) by millions of other human beings.
- If I am curious and value my feelings, I will learn how to improve my life.
- I don't have to do anything with my feelings; I simply can have them.
- There is no shame in expressing any of my feelings to others.
- I won't let others humiliate or shame me about my feelings.
- My feelings are my own, and no one can tell me what I should or shouldn't feel.
- It's OK to share my feelings, even if it makes other people uncomfortable.

- I take complete responsibility for my feelings and expect others to take responsibility for theirs.
- I'll try to manage my own feelings and expect others to manage theirs.
- No one can make me feel anything.
- I can learn how to both contain and express my feelings as need be.
- I give myself permission to feel whatever feelings surface within me.
- My feelings need not be a burden to other people.

There are practically infinite permutations of the above beliefs. Some you might already agree with, and others may seem shocking or wrong to you. For example, if you grew up with parents who devalued or neglected your feelings, you might truly believe that no one cares what you feel and that sharing your feelings with others will place an undue burden on them or end up with your being rebuffed and humiliated. In fact, you may have survived your childhood emotionally by not sharing your feelings with your parents because you knew you would be knocking on a door where no one was home.

However, your parents are only two people in a world populated by billions! Everyone else is not necessarily like them. There are healthy people who *will* value your feelings and eagerly want to hear them, people who will be honored to provide you with comfort and solace. If you believe that people don't want to know how you feel, you'll find those exact kind of people because the situation will feel familiar. If you believe that people are willing and able to care for your feelings, you'll seek people who are good listeners and emotional caretakers. And you will find them!

What can I do when I have an uncomfortable feeling?

You don't have to *do* anything when you have an uncomfortable feeling, despite any messages you may have gotten from our action-oriented culture, from your parents or TV or the movies, from the "leaders" of our society, or from how truly difficult it is to simply *be* with feelings rather than finding something to *do* with or about them. When you look at all the paths people take to distract themselves from being with their feelings—drinking, drugs, talking, sleeping, eating, shopping, exercising, obsessing, working, ruminating, blaming, arguing—it would be perfectly natural to believe that feelings were in great need of doing something with them.

However, the best thing you can do with a feeling is often nothing at all, a sterling example of how less can be more. The goal is for you to learn to *be* with your feelings, which means acknowledging and experiencing them, allowing them do the work they're meant to do, then letting them go. Remember that their purpose is to educate and inform you about your internal world.

Feelings surface and disappear, erupt and dissipate. The only thing you need to do is be open to this natural movement, the flow of feelings. This kind of passivity can be excruciatingly hard work if you are an action-oriented, go-get-'em, problem-solving kind of person, or if you feel threatened when you're not in strict control of your internal and external environment. However, your fear or discomfort arises from ignorance about the true purpose of feelings—the transmission of data. So the idea that you need to do something with a feeling is erroneous, unhelpful, and ultimately unhealthy.

Do you feel you must do something every time you get a new piece of information from your environment via your senses? My guess is that you simply take in the information without feeling compelled to take action with every single sensation you experience. Do you run away every time you smell something burning, or do you sometimes enjoy the musky smoke of a fire in your hearth or of chicken sizzling on the grill? Yes, sometimes it is appropriate to take action, but often it's enough to simply absorb the sensation and let it be.

What are some good ways to be with feelings?

Now you're on the right track, asking the right question. Learning to be with your feelings is a skill that takes practice. Many people feel overwhelmed the minute they notice a pinch of emotional unease. They don't know how to handle the feeling and, therefore, want to get rid of it ASAP. By learning to manage your feelings, you'll feel less frightened and overwhelmed by them and be better able to cope when they pay you an inevitable visit. Moreover, if there's any key to "normal" eating for disordered eaters, it's learning the skill of emotional management.

Follow these steps every time you feel an uncomfortable or painful feeling. Keep practicing until the process becomes as automatic as driving your car or getting ready for bed. Remember the marble on the hill of sand and the fact that neural pathways are being built whenever you repeat an action. Practicing these steps will lead you to exactly where you want to be—simply *being* with your feelings.

Steps for managing emotions

1. **Acknowledge** that you have an uncomfortable or painful feeling.

   - When you sense the slightest jolt or murmur of a feeling, STOP what you are doing (at least internally) and pay immediate attention. Information is incoming.

   - Notice where in your body you feel the emotion (for example, intestines, chest, throat, jaw, eyes, heart).

   - Suspend judgment about your emotional unease and substitute compassion and curiosity. Do not move on to step 2 until you've stopped judging yourself.

2. **Identify** what you are feeling.

   - Ask yourself the name of the feeling or describe it in a few words.

   - Be as specific as possible in capturing the feeling (that is, *betrayed* rather than *angry*, *bereft* rather than *sad*, *disappointed* rather than *upset*, *rejected* rather than *hurt*).

   - If you identify the feeling as anger, dig deeper. Anger is usually a secondary feeling that covers, protects, or defends against a more vulnerable one such as helplessness, fear, hurt, or abandonment.

   - If you're feeling a number of similar feelings, identify as many as you can. For example, you may be feeling disappointed, rejected, and shocked all at once.

   - If you're feeling conflicting feelings, resist the urge to erase one of them from your emotional blackboard. Give yourself permission to have feelings, and identify them accurately, both sad and relieved, both frightened and excited.

3. **Experience** what you are feeling.

- Prepare yourself for experiencing sensations of discomfort or pain with a reminder that you're doing something healthy for yourself and that experiencing this feeling will prevent you from acting out with food.

- Ask yourself these important questions relating to your beliefs:

  - Why am I afraid to feel this feeling?

  - What do I fear will happen if I allow myself to feel?

  - Am I afraid that the feeling will never stop?

  - Am I afraid I'll go crazy, be overwhelmed, or get depressed?

  - Am I afraid that the feeling could somehow kill me?

- Reframe your irrational beliefs about ending up in the hospital or taking your life and reassure yourself that nothing bad will happen by experiencing this feeling because, just as feelings come, they will go.

- Gently push aside your resistance to the feeling and accept that a feeling is paying you a visit. Simply invite it in, nothing more. Let *it* dictate any action you take—bawl your heart out, rock or hug yourself, curl up in a fetal ball. Don't hold anything back.

- Allow the feeling to stay until it's ready to go. Remind yourself that it will subside.

4. **Recover** from the feeling.

- When the feeling has subsided, praise yourself to the skies for having survived your experience. Don't worry about whether or when it will return. Stay present.

- Notice if you have any lingering judgments or secondary emotions about having had the feeling. (That is, are you angry that you felt dejected? Do you pity yourself for feeling lonely? Are you ashamed that you felt jealous?)

- Let go of judgments and remind yourself that feelings simply *are* and that you had a good reason for feeling as you did.

- Etch this experience into your memory so that you will recall surviving this feeling. This will reassure you that you can bear it next time it visits.

5. (Optional) **Deal** with the feeling.

- Observe whether this feeling is common and frequent in your life. Ask yourself if there's anything you can do to change your behavior to avoid having this feeling. (That is, are you engaged in voluntary or involuntary suffering?) Sometimes the answer is yes, as in the case of allowing people to take advantage of you. If you change your behavior and no longer allow them to use you, you won't feel used by them. Sometimes the answer is no, as in the case of missing a loved one. Feeling sad is a natural part of breaking attachments, and you must learn to bear this kind of unpleasantness if you are going to continue making meaningful connections.

- Pay careful attention to how feelings are created from your belief system. Decide if the belief beneath a feeling is healthy and rational. For example, if you don't receive a return phone call from a friend when you expected it, you may feel rejected or neglected (or both). These feelings may come from your belief that you're not lovable or that you can't keep close friends. Change the belief to thinking that your friend might be busy or may have forgotten to call because she's overwhelmed, and you'll be less likely to feel personally hurt by her.

- If you feel a need to take action, don't make a decision about what to do in the heat of the moment. Instead, promise yourself that in order to avoid the feeling you've just experienced, you will in the future consider changing your behavior by doing any or all of the following:
  - Share your feelings
  - Assert your needs
  - Confront, distance from, or avoid someone
  - Refuse to participate in an unhealthy relationship or situation

These steps for experiencing and managing feelings may constitute the most important section of this book for two reasons. First, managing feelings is something that will help you improve your life in ways that go beyond your desire to be a "normal" eater. Emotional management is an essential component of healthy well-being. And, second, handling your feelings effectively is your primary tool for achieving a functional, enjoyable relationship with food. I promise you, if you're deeply into experiencing a feeling with true acceptance and without judgment, food will be the last thing on your mind.

Are you saying that if I end my abusive relationship with food, my life will automatically improve?

Unfortunately, there are no guarantees in life. However, based on my own and my clients' and students' experiences, the odds are excellent that your life will change exponentially for the better when you stop depending on food to help you through emotional turbulence. Knowing that you can trust your body and manage your food intake is a huge achievement and a natural consequence of handling your emotions effectively.

When you no longer use food (eating or avoiding it) to manage your emotions, you may feel a temporary vacuum in your life. You have cleaned out a messy area of your mind and left a big empty space, a gaping hole. If you start refilling the space with junk, your mind will soon be as packed as it was before your cleaning spree. If you replace disordered eating with shopping, drinking, exercising, or any other addictive activity that distances you from feeling, you'll have switched your path, but your destination will remain the same: denial and self-estrangement. However, if you're very selective about what you place in that empty area, your mind and your life will be enriched.

Only when you can stop your disordered eating and form a healthier relationship with food will you begin to understand what's missing in your life and what will bring you lasting joy and contentment. Ask yourself what you're lacking: peace or excitement, meaning or frivolity, connection or disconnection, or a healthy balance of all these. The trick is to sit with an open heart and mind until the answer comes along—hobbies, new buddies, travel, a better job, relocating, sprucing yourself up, taking time off, pacing yourself better.

For example, if you end up frequently disappointed by your partner and have been using food obsessions to hide from this fact, you may initially find acknowledging your feelings quite unsettling. However, only when you allow yourself to feel the disappointment will you be able to take steps toward changing your relationship—or your partner. When you stop acting out around food every time you're lonely and begin to sit with the isolation and disconnection, you'll discover the steps you need to build more connections or deepen the intimacy of your current ones. Once you stop "taking care" of your feelings by eating too much or too little, you'll open the door to finding authentic, infinite, lasting ways to be good to your favorite person—yourself!

The amount and kind of changes you make will depend on how deeply you allow yourself to feel the intensity of your feelings, how strongly you're motivated to change, and what kind of risk taker you are. The drawbacks of disordered eating are all too familiar; you've been there and done that a hundred times before—obsessing about your weight, feeling out of control or exercising rigid control, compromising your health, distancing yourself from your body, and distracting yourself from uncomfortable feelings. The risks of giving up disordered eating and making a happy, healthy life for yourself, however, are unknown. In the process of trying to reach your goals, you may experience even more unhappiness. But if you don't distract yourself with food issues and if you keep learning from your mistakes and taking risks, you'll eventually create a better life for yourself.

7

"NORMAL" EATING BEHAVIORS

Can You Really Teach an Old Mouth New Tricks?

Building emotional muscle and stamina, that is, learning to sit with intense feelings for as long as it takes for them to pass, is only one of the ways to move toward "normal" eating. The second, as you know, is transforming your *beliefs* about food, eating, weight, and your body to align with how "normal" eaters think. And the third, of course, is changing your *behavior*. How "normal" eaters behave around food may seem mysterious and magical, but that's because you don't have the skills they use unconsciously to eat "normally." It's important to remember that you have skills in other areas they lack. And that you *can* learn what they already know!

What's the main difference between the eating behaviors of compulsive/emotional, restrictive, and "normal" eaters?

The major difference between restrictive, compulsive/emotional, and "normal" eaters is that chronic overeating or undereating is predominantly shame-based and riddled with intrapsychic conflict, while "normal" eating is pretty much only about food, appetites, and sensory pleasure. In compulsive/emotional eating, shame and internal conflicts about being or becoming fat and eating too much or the "wrong" foods generate behavior that includes disconnecting from what you're eating, eating to stuff down feelings, disengaging your body from the feeding process, detaching your mind from physical sensation, and eating rapidly so that food—the source of the shame—disappears quickly. If you can't make your shameful self vanish, then you have to make the food disappear instead.

In restrictive eating, shame about unease around food and fear of becoming fat produce behaviors that include feeling the need to be in control at all times around food, setting rigid limits with food quantities, not eating or not eating enough, eating in such a way as to pretend you are enjoying food when you aren't, eating only the "right" foods, valuing quantity over quality, tying your self-worth to how much or how little you've eaten, and constantly making judgments about your food intake.

Both compulsive overeaters and undereaters are often intensely ashamed of their helplessness and powerlessness around food and what they believe to be their unhealthy *need* for food, which can border on desperation. This feeling of shame about needing may have been learned in childhood. If your parents were unable to meet your ordinary emotional and physical childhood needs, you may have learned to believe that these needs were unusual or excessive and that you should be ashamed of them. Helplessness and powerlessness need not necessarily lead to feeling shame, but they frequently do when we're taught that these feelings are unacceptable. If you were chronically shamed, degraded, ignored, humiliated, neglected, or otherwise abused when you expressed valid needs, especially emotional ones, then shame may be an automatic response to having needs. Now as an adult, you have another chance to take a look at this pattern and perhaps change your belief, based on your new perspective: needs are normal, not shameful. You have the right to have needs and to make your needs known.

"Normal" eaters simply don't associate shame with eating, although they may have other shame-based behaviors or addictions. "Normal" eaters feel no threat around food. They have faith in their body signals regarding their appetite, and they don't imagine that people are judging what they eat or don't eat. Shame has no place in their attitude toward food and, therefore, they eat with a sense of freedom that restrictive or compulsive/emotional eaters only dream about.

Remember the triadic link among feelings, beliefs, and behaviors? If you *believe* that you're not entitled to eat freely, that eating is a shameful behavior, two things happen: 1) You eat freely and feel ashamed or prevent yourself from eating freely to avoid feeling ashamed. Either way, the focus is not on food but on your current or anticipated emotional state. 2) Because your goal of warding off shame has nothing to do with food and everything to do with feeling, your behaviors interrupt the natural connection between your body and food.

What exactly are the behaviors involved in "normal" eating?

You already know what the rules of "normal" eating are—and what are rules but ways of governing behavior? The rules define the basic ways in which "normal" eaters think about and react concerning food. Soon you'll learn how to fill in the finer details to complete the picture. Before we move on to the specific behaviors that "normal" eaters use every day, let's review the rules:

1. Eat when you are hungry or have a craving for a specific food.
2. Choose foods that you believe will satisfy you.
3. Stay connected to your body and eat with awareness and enjoyment.
4. Stop eating when you are full or satisfied.

Each of these four rules has a set of skills that you need to learn. And each set of skills or behaviors can be acquired through attention, patience, and practice. The main difficulty is that your life is not a clean slate being written upon. Instead, it's a slate that's already been scribbled all over. The outdated, dysfunctional, messages will have to be erased so that new, improved ones can take their place. This means that while you're learning new skills, you're simultaneously unlearning old ones.

The next section lists the skills required to live by each rule of "normal" eating. The skills need not be acquired in any particular order, but they all need to be practiced over and over until they become part of your automatic eating and thinking-about-food repertoire. "Normal" eaters developed these skills naturally in childhood, and even they don't practice every one of them every time they eat. However, because they know they possess these skills, they are able to call on them when the need arises.

For example, one of the skills for staying connected to your body is to eat only when you're relaxed. Obviously, "normal" eaters eat sometimes when they're tense, upset, stressed, or in a hurry. Even so, they're able to stay connected with physical sensations because they've had years of practice and because the connection is automatic and unconscious. I doubt that many air traffic controllers munched on veggie wraps as they were being taught to do their job; however, I'm fairly certain that many now feel comfortable enough with their aviation knowledge and experience to enjoy a snack while at the controls in a nonemergency situation.

RULE 1: Eat when you are hungry or have a craving for a specific food.

To live by this rule, you must be able to:

- Identify hunger
- Allow yourself to feel your hunger
- Accept hunger as natural and beneficial
- Differentiate hunger from thirst, tiredness, and other body sensations
- Postpone eating until you are moderately hungry
- Give yourself permission to eat if you are hungry
- Identify a craving for a particular food
- Differentiate craving from the urge to eat for emotional reasons
- Give yourself permission to eat what your body craves

- Say yes to food appropriately
- Say no to food appropriately
- Tolerate the anxiety that will likely arise when you try to respond authentically from internal cues about your hunger rather than following arbitrary external guidelines
- Refrain from negative judgments about hunger and craving

RULE 2: Choose foods that you believe will satisfy you.

To live by this rule, you must to be able to:

- Eliminate judgmental beliefs about foods being "good" or "bad"
- Clear your mind of any *should*, *must*, *need to*, *shouldn't*, and *can't* ideas about what to eat except if you are physically allergic to foods
- Feel comfortable saying yes to foods you desire or crave
- Feel comfortable saying no to foods you dislike or don't want
- Refrain from counting calories or fat grams and measuring or weighing food
- Refrain from evaluating food strictly from a nutritional standpoint
- Stay in the moment without focusing on what you've already eaten or will be eating later on
- Identify your body's messages about what it wants to eat
- Have patience with the time it takes to select food that will be satisfying
- Eat without guilt, shame, fear, or anxiety

- Believe that only you and no one else in the world knows what you want to eat
- Look forward to food and eating as pleasurable
- Be comfortable sending your food back in a restaurant if it doesn't taste right, and requesting something else
- Hurt someone's feelings if your body says it doesn't want a particular food
- Make food choices without seeking others' approval

RULE 3: Stay connected to your body and eat with awareness.
To live by this rule, you must be able to:

- Remain present to the physical sensations of eating
- Refrain from feeling guilty or ashamed about what you are eating
- Avoid tensing up while you are eating
- Postpone eating until you are relaxed enough to enjoy it
- Create a time and space for yourself that is conducive to eating
- Avoid being distracted by what others are eating or talking about or by preoccupation with other concerns (such as work, relationships, etc.)
- Taste every bite of what you are eating
- Eat slowly, take small bites, and pause frequently while eating
- Ask yourself frequently whether you're enjoying what you're eating
- Ask yourself frequently whether you're still hungry

- Look at your food often and see what's left on your plate
- Refrain from eating on the run
- Turn off your mind to chatter about food and tune in to physical feelings

RULE 4: Stop eating when you are full or satisfied.

To live by this rule, you must be able to:

- Stay connected to your body and eat with awareness
- Identify the physical and mental sensations that tell you that your stomach is full
- Identify the physical and mental sensations that tell you that both your body and mind are satisfied
- Eat without feeling guilt and shame
- Give your brain enough time to register fullness and satiation
- Tolerate the feeling of deprivation that may come from saying "No more" to food
- Feel comfortable leaving food on your plate
- Feel comfortable throwing or giving away food
- Feel comfortable eating all the food on your plate and more if you are still hungry
- Tolerate the anxiety that may come from arriving at fullness or satisfaction
- Turn off your thoughts of food when full or satisfied and redirect your thinking toward other things
- Believe that you can have more of what you are eating at another time
- Be in touch with sensations of "enough"

I hope you're not feeling overwhelmed by all you need to learn and that you're not putting undue pressure on yourself to acquire all these new skills instantly. You probably wish you'd learned them yesterday and are thinking that you would give practically anything to awaken with them tomorrow. But let's be real. You're not going to become a "normal" eater overnight, no matter how desperate or impatient you feel.

If you've slipped into thinking that you can magically throw yourself into overdrive and practice night and day to develop these skills more quickly, or if you are feeling hopeless that you'll ever manage the totality of the eating behaviors listed above, go back and reread Chapter 2: The Rules of Change. When you've finished, work on retooling your thinking about patience and pacing yourself, both of which you'll need for the long haul. The more you work on developing healthy, positive beliefs about change and progress, the easier it will be to learn the skills of "normal" eating.

What exercises can I use to practice the skills needed to eat "normally"?

At your next eating experience you can begin using exercises that will help you acquire the skills needed to become a "normal" eater. At first you might feel strange and uncomfortable, and you may be tempted to resist doing them. They're not meant to be fun (though some may be), and you can find a million excuses not to do them, including forgetting that you want to do them at all. This is natural because the behaviors embodied in these exercises are not only unfamiliar but antithetical to your current eating practices. However, if you want to become a "normal" eater, you'll have to do the work. There is no other way.

If you are in a welcoming frame of mind to do these exercises, you'll feel curious, upbeat, and maybe even a little excited about learning new ways to approach food. If you stay open to learning about what behaviors prevent you from eating "normally," you'll discover a great deal about your internal barriers. Use the exercises to retrain yourself to become a "normal" eater. Return to them whenever you relapse into compulsive, emotional, or restrictive eating. These practices will ground you in your body and help you reconnect to physical sensations. After a while, they will move from being conscious to unconscious, and you'll be surprised and thrilled when you use them without realizing it.

A side note about these exercises. I was taught to ski by learning to exaggerate the movements that are used in skiing. To make a turn, I would take the weight off my uphill ski by thrusting my body upward as if I were shooting toward the sky. To transfer my weight to my downhill ski at the end of a turn, I would bend my knees and crouch low. To learn to keep my body weight forward and my arms parallel and out in front of me, I would pretend I was holding a dinner tray. At first I felt self-conscious and somewhat ridiculous using such dramatic movements, but after a lesson my body remembered the exaggerated lifts and crouches precisely *because* they had been overemphasized. My instructor never suggested that I ski with such pronounced postures forever, but he understood that to learn, a body needs a strong physical memory.

Here are some exercises that will help you learn the skills needed for each rule of "normal" eating. However, an exercise to help you tune in to your hunger before you eat may also help you stay connected to your body while you're eating and then help you stop eating when you're full or satisfied. Some exercises are strictly internal, and you can do them without anyone knowing that you're hard at work. Others require that you be in a space where you feel comfortable eating.

Exercises for Tuning In to Hunger

- At random times during the day, ask yourself if you're hungry and give your hunger a number (10 equals famished, and 0 equals not a bit hungry). If you think this will be a difficult exercise to remember, set an alarm (a watch with an alarm is helpful) to remind you. The exercise isn't complete until you've come up with a number.

- At a time when you're not hungry, prepare or take out food that you think will be potentially satisfying when you are hungry. Periodically look at and sniff the food while doing a hunger check. Notice what happens to your hunger in the presence of the food. Does the mere sight of food cause you to salivate, making you want to gobble it up then and there? Or does it terrify you? If you're a compulsive eater, what do you need to think, feel, and do to delay eating until you're hungry enough? If you're a restrictive eater, how can you reorient your thoughts and feelings when you're hungry but find yourself resisting food?

- Every time you think about food, ask yourself how hungry you are. Try to gauge how often you think about food when you aren't hungry. Is it more often than you think about food when you are hungry? What would you be thinking about if you didn't constantly have food on your mind?

- Try forcing yourself to become hungry and see what happens. Can you come up with the physical symptoms of hunger using thought alone? Wait until you're hungry and try forcing yourself not to be. Do your hunger symptoms disappear? Decide to let your body rule in the matter of hunger.

- Every time you're ready to eat, make sure you know what hunger range you're in: slightly, moderately, or very. Don't allow yourself to take a lick or a bite without identifying a range.

- Note exactly where in your body you feel hunger. Be able to count off on one hand your body's signals that you need food.

- Occasionally force yourself to eat when you're not at all hungry and notice how your body responds. What are the signals it gives you to stop eating?

- Wait until you're starving to eat and notice how your body reacts. What are the signals it gives you to eat more or more quickly?

Exercises for Tuning In to a Craving

- At random times during the day, check in with yourself and notice if you have any food cravings. Do you never crave foods? How come? Do you squelch your cravings because you're scared you'll act on them? Do you have the same cravings over and over? What are the circumstances?

- Whenever you're around food, get into the habit of asking yourself whether you crave it. When you pass a bakery, ice cream parlor, juice bar, candy store, Chinese restaurant, fruit and vegetable market, or fast food restaurant, check in with yourself to see if you have a desire for what you see and smell.

- When you have a craving, stop whatever you're doing and pay attention. Imagine yourself eating the food and notice whether the fantasy enhances, diminishes, or satisfies your craving.

- Look through a cookbook and note the recipes that ring your chimes. Just flip through pages quickly and react. Let your body say yes or no automatically without judgment or interfering thoughts.

- Notice where in your body you sense a craving and exactly how your body signals what food it desires.

- Force yourself to "want" a certain food and notice how your body reacts.

- When you have a craving, force your body to "not want" that food and notice how it responds. Do cravings come and go? If you're used to saying no to cravings, try giving in to them more often. If you always give in to them, see what happens when you don't.

- Assess your cravings as mild, moderate, or intense. Would you enjoy the food more if you craved it moderately or intensely rather than mildly?

- Practice saying yes to food by glancing in the mirror during noneating times and saying aloud with a broad smile, "Yes, I'd love some, thank you."

Exercises for Choosing Satisfying Foods

- Practice the craving and hunger exercises so that your body gets into the habit of giving you a response to food.

- If you don't know what you want to eat at home, flip through the pages of a cookbook to see if anything sparks your interest. If you're near a bookstore, before eating out, find the cookbook section and thumb through recipes to see what strikes your fancy.

- Test your taste buds with fantasies of foods—sweet, sour, salty, bitter, spicy, etc.

- When selecting food, imagine what you will feel like: a) while you're eating it, and b) after you've eaten it. Do you love foods that don't love you? The goal is to enjoy your food and have the delicious feeling linger after the food is gone. This is meant to be a physical exercise, not a mental one, about feelings of guilt or shame. Notice that some foods you love might disagree with you by giving you gas, nausea, indigestion, or heartburn.

- Practice saying yes to cravings you have and no to thoughts that aren't actually cravings.

- Approach food with neutrality, without labeling it good or bad.

- In restaurants, choose an alternate menu selection in case your first choice isn't available. You'll be getting double the practice in selecting satisfying foods and, if you don't get your first choice, you won't feel bitterly disappointed.

Exercises for Staying Connected to Your Body and Eating with Awareness

- Practice eating without any distractions during at least one meal a day. The more times you practice this exercise, the faster you will reestablish connections between eating and your body. By the way, no distractions means no TV, radio, talking on the phone, computer work, any other kind of work, checking snail mail or e-mail, reading, or leafing through a magazine. No distractions means nada, niet, zilch, zip, zero.

- When you're eating, set a timer to go off every 3 or 4 minutes, reminding you to ask yourself if you're enjoying your food.

- If you generally eat fast, slow down. Set a timer to go off 10 minutes later than the time it usually takes you to eat, and stretch out your eating until it rings.

- If you generally eat slowly to avoid the end of the eating experience, try picking up the pace to a more moderate speed and see how you feel.

- Put down your utensil after every three or four bites and pause to look at your food. Notice how much you've eaten or not eaten. Use this pause to ask yourself if you're enjoying your food. If you're not, figure out why.

- If you're used to taking huge bites, take smaller bites before swallowing.

- If you're used to prolonged chewing, stop chewing sooner.

- Wait until one bite is completely swallowed before taking another.

- If you're a gobbler, let every bite of food sit on your tongue for about 3 seconds to make sure you get a strong hit of flavor. Pretend you're being paid extremely handsomely to extract every bit of flavor from every mouthful.

- Eat an entire meal with your fingers.

- Close your eyes when you eat and focus exclusively on your mouth and the route food takes to your stomach. Imagine that this path is highlighted in gold.

- Take three deep breaths between every mouthful and sigh in exaggerated satisfaction from the exquisite pleasure of eating. If there's no pleasure, why eat?

- Scan your body for tension every time you begin to eat and then once or twice while eating. If you feel tension, stop eating immediately and relax the area until the tension is gone. Then resume eating.

- Remind yourself that the quality of food is more important than the quantity.

Exercises for Tuning In to Fullness

- After every mouthful or two, ask yourself if you still have signs of hunger. If the answer is yes, keep eating. If no, then you're full and it's time to quit.

- Recall the exact physical feeling you have when you've overeaten. Describe it aloud or write down what it feels like. Similarly, describe the sensations of feeling nicely full. Notice the difference.

- If you're still hungry or still enjoying what you're eating, notice if you're upset by the fear that you're eating too much.

- Get up two or three times while you're eating and go into another room. Reach deeply inside yourself and ask if you're still hungry.

- If you've stopped eating and left the table before you are genuinely full, experiment to see what happens if you return and continue eating.

- Stop eating when you're still a little hungry and notice any emotions that surface. Eat slightly past full, stop, and notice the emotions that surface. Really stuff yourself and notice your emotions. Compare your reactions.

- Practice sliding your chair away from the table when you're full by pushing against the table with your hands. Does being physically farther away from food make a difference in your emotions about being finished?

- If you're a compulsive eater, focus on how little food it actually takes to fill you up.

- If you're a restrictive eater, focus on how much food it takes to feel truly full.

- If you feel sad that you're full and ready to stop eating, allow yourself a moment of grief. Cry if you need to, or simply make a sad face. Stopping eating can feel like a loss, and it's healthy to acknowledge the intensity of any feeling.

- Notice how the sensations of getting full—your stomach feeling enlarged and pressing against your waistband— can trick you into thinking you are fat. Gently push your fear of fat out of your decisions about fullness.

- If you're full, picture yourself stopping eating and either putting away the food for another time or throwing it out.

- Practice saying no to food by glancing in the mirror at noneating times and saying aloud with a broad smile, "No, thanks, I'm finished now."

Exercises for Tuning In to Satisfaction

- Pretend you're explaining to a person from another planet how it feels to be satisfied by food. Give them a detailed account of how you know you're satisfied.

- After every mouthful or two, ask yourself if you're satisfied yet. If the answer is no, keep eating, by all means. If yes, then it's time to stop.

- Eat your favorite food very slowly and count how many bites it takes for you to be satisfied. Don't push yourself to eat fewer or more bites. Try this exercise with the same food during different times of the day and on different days. Try the exercise with your five favorite foods.

- Try to find the peak moment when you know you're satisfied. If you were taking a snapshot, you'd wait for that special instant, then focus and click. You can capture that same feeling by waiting until you have found the perfect time to stop eating.

- Put a sign on your table that reads, "Am I satisfied yet?"

- Stop eating before you're satisfied and notice how you feel emotionally. Stop when you've eaten beyond satisfaction and notice how you feel.

- Once you're satisfied, picture yourself stopping eating and either putting away the food for another time or throwing it out.

- Set a timer for every 3 or 4 minutes and when it goes off, ask yourself, "Am I satisfied yet?"
- Reflect on whether it takes more or less food than you thought to be satisfied. Which is more important to you—satisfaction or fullness?
- If you never or rarely allow yourself to feel satisfied by food, keep inching your way forward until you reach that yummy moment.
- Remind yourself as you eat that you have the right to enjoy food and feel satisfied by it.

How can I learn how to really trust my mind and body around food?

Whether you're working on saying yes to food, no to food, or trying to get the right balance, learning to trust yourself takes time. Because your mind and body have betrayed you so often in the past, you may fear that you can never trust them. But a little trust will build more trust; each experience of satisfying yourself with food will build those neural pathways and make you more likely to trust your mind and body cues the next time. If you have an all-or-nothing attitude about trust—*I can trust myself completely,* or *I cannot trust myself at all around food*—remind yourself that there are shades of gray and consider terms such as *a little*, *rarely*, *a good deal*, *a great deal*, and *often*.

What you believed yesterday about food, eating, weight, and your body produced yesterday's feelings and behaviors. What you believe today will produce an entirely new set of feelings and behaviors. One reason to take the risk of trusting yourself more around food now is that your thinking and feelings are changing. Remember, transform the beliefs, and your feelings and behavior will change too. You can trust yourself more now because you're thinking more rationally, and rational thinking leads to healthy feelings and behavior.

Try experimenting. Whether you've decided to eat more or less, see if you can sit with the guilt or anxiety that comes from picking up your fork or putting it down. Notice how terrifying and intense the feelings are. Hold on to your chair, take deep breaths, count to ten, do whatever you have to do to let the feeling rise and fall. *I cannot underscore strongly enough how the inability to bear pain and discomfort is at the root of dysfunctional eating.* If you've survived the feeling, give yourself a round of applause. You're on your way to trusting yourself more.

Remember, your terrors are nothing but a memory of what actually happened or what you feared would happen in childhood. At present they're only the unwanted, unhelpful product of an overactive imagination. No matter how anxious or guilty you feel, eat when you're hungry or have a craving, eat what you want, and stop when you're full or satisfied. Then wait and see what bad thing happens. NOTHING BAD HAPPENS! Not one damn thing, other than feeling uneasy. The food police exist only in your mind. Nothing terrible will happen if you eat, and nothing bad will happen if you stop eating.

The only way you will know I'm speaking the absolute, rock-bottom truth is by experiencing this yourself, by sitting with anxiety, guilt, shame, and fear until you realize that you're still OK. If you do this over and over (and over and over), you'll gradually find release from the anxiety, fear, shame, guilt, and other uneasy feelings you associated with the activity of eating. It's not enough to work on your beliefs. You need to be comfortable with your feelings.

Something wonderful will happen when you learn to tolerate discomfort around food and let your mind and body respond authentically: you'll slowly begin to trust yourself. Trust comes from knowing that you can be depended on to do what is best for yourself. It can't be learned by listening to what others tell you, no matter how important these people are in your life or how well meaning they are. It can only develop over time, by listening to your deepest wisdom about yourself. Trust grows from your own experience: *I did it once, so I can do it again.* Once you have allowed yourself to sit with a difficult feeling or engage in an unfamiliar behavior, you can do it a second time and a third. The more you do it, the easier it will get, until you know that you can trust yourself because you are courageous and have your best interests at heart.

8

CARING FOR YOURSELF

*You Mean Do Unto Myself As I Would
Do Unto Others?*

What if you viewed chronic overeating or undereating not as a disorder, sickness, condition, character weakness, tragic flaw, or illness, but as your very best effort to deal with your life? What if eating or denying yourself food has been nothing more than a misguided attempt to take care of yourself? What if you didn't look at disordered eating as your worst problem, but as your best solution to date?

There's a psychological principle that maintains that you're always doing the best you can. Even when you're doing poorly, the principle holds true. For example, you might wish to do a better job of managing your eating, but given your history and who you are at this point in time, a mediocre or poor job might be the best you can do right now. Saying that you're doing the best you can in no way implies that you cannot, will not, or should not ever do better. It's neither a condemnation of your present nor a prognosis for your future, neither a criticism nor a judgment of your efforts, abilities, or potential. It's merely a statement of fact, a description of where you are right now. If you could do better, you would. It's as simple as that. Moreover, if you desire to do better, it's probable that you *will,* and that's something to be hopeful about. Paradoxically, accepting that you're doing your best right now (and have been all along) is a powerful tool for actually doing better tomorrow.

This is a hard concept to wrap your mind around, I know. I'm used to having clients and students challenge me when I tell them that they (or someone else) may not be doing the best they *ever* can but that they're doing their best right *now.* I'll understand if you're thinking, Of course I could do better; I'm just not trying hard enough; How can this be the best I can do? I refuse to cop out and accept this as my best. What I ask is that instead of challenging this new concept, you try aiming your energy toward understanding that even though your best might not be good enough for you or others, it's the highest level of functioning you're able to achieve at the moment.

So, you might be wondering, what does accepting that I'm doing my best have to do with food and taking care of myself? The answer is that moving toward or away from food has somehow turned into a major way you've learned to take care of yourself physically and emotionally. It's neither healthy nor effective, but it's the best approach you've found to date. There are reasons that you use your relationship with food to take care of yourself, and you're fortunate that you have the ability (alone or with help) to reflect back on your childhood and discover them.

Remember, what you learned yesterday resulted in who you are today; what you learn today will result in who you are tomorrow.

Before exploring how and where self-care is learned, it's important to recognize what self-care is. First and foremost, it's a reflection of self-worth. The quality of self-care you practice is predicated on how much you value yourself. In general, if you value something highly, you take good care of it. Conversely, if you don't think too much of something, you probably won't put much effort into taking care of it. This concept is as true for people as it is for material objects. The care you take is directly related to your perception of worth.

How did I learn about self-care?

Let's say that your parents never showed you how to brush your teeth correctly, which they should have, and that you're still doing a pretty sloppy job of it. You might not even realize that you're not brushing long enough, or that you're brushing too hard or in the wrong direction. You might just breeze along, brushing your teeth as you always have until someone, perhaps your dentist or hygienist, advises you differently.

Similarly, if your parents had an unhealthy relationship with food, they probably unconsciously modeled this dysfunction for you as a child. Even if you weren't abused or neglected in your early years, if your parents turned toward or away from food to cope with *their* problems, you would believe that these big, powerful, significant people knew exactly what they were doing. Why wouldn't you assume that they were right and strive to copy them? The fact is, it was perfectly natural and normal for you to accept what your parents did as appropriate self-care and for you to continue the same behavior without giving it a second thought.

Our knowledge about self-care comes to us in the same way as our learning about beliefs. It's not taught as a special subject, but it is subtly woven into the fabric of our young lives. We learn by watching how our parents or caretakers take care of themselves: monkey see, monkey do. We also learn through the way we are taken care of and through what we are told and taught about good self-care, whether our parents practice it or not. The fact is that our training occurs long before we have any idea that we are being schooled.

Doesn't self-care mean being self-centered and self-indulgent?

Absolutely not. The misconception that taking excellent care of yourself means that you are either selfish or self-indulgent was probably learned in your childhood. Your parents didn't mean to confuse you, but they were probably confused themselves about what healthy caretaking entails.

Let's start with a functional family care model and then see where your family may have run into trouble. In healthy family caretaking, each adult takes care of himself or herself *and* their partner, more or less in balance. The family functions on the principle of mutuality: I do not have to hurt myself to take care of your needs, and you do not have to hurt yourself to take care of mine. Your needs and my needs are equally important, and both can be met. This model promotes interdependence. For example, I'll do what you want this time, and you do what I want next time. Both of our needs are valued and considered. The focus is not on competition or tit for tat, but on the recognition that what goes around comes around and on overall enhancement of the family unit. Members of a functional family know that everyone benefits when each individual, as well as the family as a whole, all receive high quality care.

In a dysfunctional family, the assumption is that in every dyad (mother-father, parent-child), only one person's needs can get met. Instead of a model of mutuality, this is a model of mutual exclusion. On a consistent basis, one (or more) family member's needs are attended to, while others' needs are ignored or brushed aside. The numerous dysfunctional permutations of this model include: mother neglects herself and puts father's needs first; mother puts herself first and neglects father's needs; father puts himself first and neglects mother's needs; father neglects himself and puts mother's needs first; mother and father both put their needs first and neglect their children's needs; father and mother neglect themselves and put their children's needs first. Do any of these models portray the way your family functioned?

Take a moment to think about how each of your parents took care of themselves, each other, and you and your siblings, if you had any. Was the model generally mutual or mutually exclusive? Was one of your parents selfish, self-centered, or self-absorbed, focusing more on their own needs and wants than on yours or anyone else's? Were both your parents like that? Did you feel that taking care of one or both of them was more important than taking care of yourself? Did they make it seem as if taking care of yourself meant you were selfish? Did they tell you this, or did you just feel it was implied? Did they suggest that taking care of you was a burden for them? Or did one or both of your parents deny their own needs while making sure to take care of everyone else's? Have you adopted a lopsided care model by which you still live today?

After decades in this field, I can honestly say that most, if not all of the disordered eaters I've known or worked with are excellent caretakers of others and poor caretakers of themselves. In fact, *caretaker* is a term that fits them to a T. Compulsive/emotional eaters often feel wickedly uncomfortable—and sometimes just plain wicked—when they take care of their own needs. Restrictive eaters are used to denying themselves pleasure in and out of the food arena, while giving their all to others. Whichever type of eater you are (and you may alternate between being an overeater and an undereater), my bet is that the caretaking you observed and experienced as a child failed to serve you and reinforce your interests. Remember, if the self-care model in your family was dysfunctional, then the thinking and behavior patterns you learned will be unhealthy as well.

Here are some unhealthy, irrational beliefs that you may have learned about taking care of yourself:

- It's better to take care of others than to take care of myself.
- Taking care of myself means I'm selfish, self-centered, self-absorbed, self-obsessed, and/or self-indulgent.
- If I take care of myself, other people will be angry, upset, hurt, or disappointed.
- I have to choose between taking care of myself and taking care of other people.
- I don't deserve to take good care of myself.
- It's too late and too hard for me to learn to take care of myself.
- I should put others' needs before mine because that's what nice people do.
- If I take care of myself now, I'll pay in spades later.

Here are some suggestions for reframing these irrational beliefs. Feel free to improvise and add your own ideas.

Irrational Belief	Rational Beliefs
It's better to take care of others than to take care of myself.	• I don't have to choose between taking care of myself and taking care of other people. • It's healthy for me to take care of myself. • I can achieve the best balance by taking care of myself *and* other people.
Taking care of myself means I'm selfish, self-centered, self-absorbed, self-obsessed, and/or self-indulgent.	• Taking care of myself means I'm healthy. • Taking good care of myself means I'm a responsible adult, and frees me from the need to be selfish, self-centered, self-absorbed, self-obsessed, or self-indulgent. • Only I can determine what it means to take care of myself.
If I take care of myself, other people will be angry, upset, hurt, or disappointed.	• Only in an unhealthy relationship could I anger, upset, or disappoint another person by taking care of myself. I want to choose healthy relationships from now on!

	• I will take care of myself, and I expect others to take care of themselves. • People who really care about me will want me to take good care of myself.
I have to choose between taking care of myself and taking care of other people.	• I am free to make my own choices about who I want to take care of. • I can take care of myself *and* other people. • When I amwell taken care of, I feel full enough to give to others.
I don't deserve to take good care of myself.	• I deserve to take good care of myself. • I'm the only one who can decide what I do and don't deserve. • Everyone deserves to take good care of themselves.
It's too late and too hard for me to learn how to take care of myself.	• Learning to take care of myself may not be as hard as I fear. • I've learned to do harder things than take care of myself. • It's never too late to learn to take care of myself. • Today is the first day of the rest of my life!

I should put others' needs before mine because that's what nice people do.	• Nice people take good care of themselves. • Only I can decide what makes me a nice person. • I can be nicer to others if I take care of myself.
If I take care of myself now, I'll pay in spades later.	• Life will reward me for taking good care of myself. • I choose to take care of myself now and always. • No one can ever take away my ability to care for myself.

If you had a childhood in which you learned irrational, unhealthy beliefs about taking care of yourself, now is the time to transform them into rational, healthy ones. Until your belief system supports a nourishing, positive view of self-care, it will be exceedingly difficult to overcome your eating problems. You may want to rush into expanding your self-care behaviors, but you'll be stymied if your belief system doesn't support the value of taking care of yourself. Once your beliefs about self-care are healthy and rational, your behavior will be far easier to change. And once you start taking better care of yourself, you won't need to ask unhealthy eating to do it for you.

What exactly do you mean by self-care or taking care of myself?

The four realms of self-care include physical, mental, psychological/emotional, and spiritual. Naturally, they are deeply intertwined and strongly affect one another, with a great deal of overlap. For instance, if you eat mainly junk foods, your body may get run down and serious health problems may ensue, preventing you from getting out and seeing friends or being able to work. Feeling isolated, your spirit might get depressed and you could come to believe that life isn't worth living. This is an extreme but not necessarily uncommon example of the interrelationships among physical, mental, psychological/emotional, and spiritual self-care.

Good self-care basically means preventing and repairing damage to oneself. It doesn't mean being good to yourself instead of, or at the expense of, others. Nor does it mean being self-centered, selfish, self-absorbed, self-indulgent, or obsessed with yourself. It's a fact of life that sometimes when you're taking care of yourself, you end up hurting others. This injury can't be helped and is a natural occurrence in relationships. I cannot emphasize this point strongly enough. Other people may get unintentionally hurt when you are taking really good care of yourself. You didn't mean to hurt them; you meant to not hurt you! No one can get through life without hurting others or being hurt. The best we all can do is try not to deliberately hurt ourselves or others.

Not everyone, of course, takes excellent care of themselves in all four self-care realms. Some people are diligent in the physical arena, exercising, getting regular checkups and medical tests, taking vitamins, keeping active, and using preventive measures to stay healthy. Other people may do well with psychological/ emotional self-care by working through problems with relationships and communication, reading self-help books, reflecting, attending therapy and transformational workshops, and sharing their feelings with friends. Others may pay special attention to mental care, enriching their minds through reading and classes, traveling extensively, challenging themselves to learn new things, staying curious about the world, and constantly looking for ways to keep mentally alert and alive. Still others may put their energy into expanding and deepening their spiritual self through self-examination, mystical, or religious classes and reading, strengthening their attachments to community or nature, and spending time in the practice of prayer, yoga, meditation, tai chi, or chi gong.

However, just as it isn't healthy to build up only one set of body muscles and ignore others, it's dangerous in the long run to focus exclusively on only one area of self-care. Yes, taking care of yourself physically or emotionally beats not taking care of yourself at all, but it also leaves you vulnerable in the areas you've neglected. Imagine the body builder or the genius with three graduate degrees, all alone with no friends. Or someone so immersed in mystical experience that she ceases taking care of her physical needs. Or the person who spends all his free time reading self-help books and going for therapy but is constantly sick and never has any fun.

What constitutes good physical self-care?

Can you tell the difference between someone who really loves her car and someone who couldn't care less about it? Of course you can. The person who's crazy about her car does everything she can to ensure that it will continue to run smoothly. She goes to a reputable mechanic for scheduled maintenance and emergency repairs. She checks her tires monthly and keeps the engine and chassis free from dirt and grime. She follows the instructions in her driver's manual and drives according to the rules of the road.

The same goes for a person. Can you spot someone who takes good physical care of herself or himself? I don't mean just outwardly. (A slick or perfectly coiffed appearance—expensive clothes and haircut, makeup, cologne, jewelry, accessories, the latest fashions—can mask a lack of genuine self-acceptance. It's like polishing your car to a high gloss while driving around on bald tires!) People who take excellent care of themselves physically are not always healthy, but they strive for good health and realize that they can do a considerable amount to contribute to it.

Good physical self-care includes but is certainly not limited to:

- Good personal hygiene—keeping yourself generally clean and washed from head to toe

- Respecting your physical limits and doing physical activities that are age appropriate

- Having routine medical and dental checkups, dental hygiene visits, blood tests, and eye exams; scheduling procedures such as a Pap smear, colonoscopy, pregnancy test, mammogram, prostate exam, and bone density scan; ordering special tests if certain conditions, such as cancer, stroke, diabetes, or heart disease, run in your family

- Attending follow-up medical visits as recommended by your doctor and following his or her advice

- Getting a second opinion if you have doubts about your diagnosis or treatment
- Not suffering with pain and discomfort because you hate doctors, dentists, or hospitals or are afraid to find out what's wrong
- Seeking nutritional counseling if appropriate
- Following the directions for taking prescribed and over-the-counter medications and using them in a responsible manner
- Eating in a way that decreases your risk of disease
- Exercising regularly with a focus on flexibility, endurance, strength, and balance
- Taking vitamin and mineral supplements daily as needed
- Investigating alternative and integrative medicine as appropriate
- Getting a good night's sleep most nights, generally about 8 hours
- Taking a nap if it helps you feel rested; not napping if it keeps you awake at night
- Learning how to manage stress effectively
- Learning how to manage your emotions effectively
- Wearing sunscreen and protective clothing
- Wearing clothing that's weather-appropriate and using an umbrella in the rain
- Not overdoing it with caffeine or alcohol
- Avoiding recreational drugs
- Never riding in a car in which the driver is alcohol- or drug-impaired

- Slowing down your pace and thinking ahead to avoid accidental injury
- Avoiding unnecessary physical risks
- Challenging your body with sports and recreational physical activity
- Wearing comfortable shoes that don't pose a risk to your balance and safety
- Avoiding clothes that are uncomfortable, too tight, or constrict your body's organs or blood flow
- Not using tobacco or tobacco products
- Staying hydrated by drinking plenty of fluids throughout the day
- Staying home from work or leaving work if you're sick
- Respecting that your body has its high energy peaks and low energy troughs

If you haven't been taking good physical care of yourself, this list might seem intimidating and overwhelming. But you don't have to follow all the suggestions right this minute. Start small by making one or two appointments or changes. Notice how you feel about taking care of your body. Does it feel a little awkward and strange? Does it feel so unfamiliar that you don't want to continue with good physical self-care? Bear with the feeling and continue to adhere to healthy practices. Too many people make the mistake of stopping good self-care because it feels unfamiliar and makes them uncomfortable. Discomfort only means that it's a new behavior and will take a little getting used to.

What constitutes good mental self-care?

Although it's impossible (and totally unnatural) to try to separate mind from body, an industrialized world tendency, when I speak of mental self-care I'm talking about your intellectual and cognitive capacities. If you don't keep your mind active, it will become sluggish and stagnant. As the old adage says, use it or lose it. Keeping your brain in gear has proven to be a preventive measure against Alzheimer's disease and general cognitive decline, and it also works prophylactically to ward off lack of confidence and self-worth!

I'm not suggesting that you become a know-it-all or permanent student simply to enhance your sense of self. I am suggesting that challenging your brain and staying intellectually engaged with and curious about the world will contribute significantly to your well-being. Keeping your brain busy with learning also makes you a more interesting person, both to yourself and others. People want to be around others who can converse intelligently on a range of subjects. Because good self-care also includes having a strong social network, staying active mentally will increase the likelihood that people will want to be a part of yours.

Good mental health care includes but is certainly not limited to:

- Keeping abreast of what's going on in your community, country, and the world
- Being able to make cogent, rational, intellectual arguments for the principles and ideas you believe in deeply; being able to back up and give evidence for your opinions
- Finding new learning opportunities through travel, books, videos, lectures, classes, workshops, and so forth

- Refraining from total reliance on tools such as calculators to do mathematical figuring
- Becoming a true master in one or two areas of knowledge or expertise
- Regularly testing your memory and keeping it sharp
- Learning new skills, hobbies, sports, and activities
- Staying open to unfamiliar ideas and ways of thinking, especially those that challenge your current views
- Using your imagination as frequently as possible
- Listening well when someone really knows what they are talking about
- Making it your business to learn about as many things as you can

A word here about following the news. I hear many people say that they don't want to know what's going on in the world because the news is generally "such a bummer." We may all feel that way at times, especially after September 11th, 2001. There *is* such a thing as news overkill, and there is no question that the media sometimes shows little interest in the sensitivities of its watchers, listeners, and readers. It's all too easy to become overwhelmed by a constant diet of disaster and tragedy.

However, good psychological/emotional self-care includes being able to tolerate the helplessness that the news often generates as well as finding ways to take action to counteract this feeling. I'm not suggesting that you turn yourself into a news junkie. I'm saying that good self-care does not include chronically sticking your head in the sand because what you hear upsets you. People who feel empowered find ways to change a situation and keep from feeling helpless. Recall Reinhold Neibuhr's "Serenity

Prayer"—learn to accept the things you cannot change and, whenever possible, take action (locally or globally) to change the things you can and make the world a better place. Nothing builds self-esteem like feeling truly empowered!

What constitutes good psychological/emotional self-care?

While the study of psychological or emotional health is not an exact science, we can make certain generalizations about it. First, people who truly value themselves take good emotional care of themselves. Remember the car analogy? To understand what constitutes good emotional self-care, we have to understand what psychological or emotional health is. And to do that, it might help to look at what it definitely is *not*.

Psychological or emotional health is not:

- Being happy, positive, confident, and upbeat all the time
- Always feeling on top of things
- Being in complete control of your life
- Being independent and never depending on others
- Having all the answers
- Being liked by everyone
- Thinking you are or trying to be perfect
- Feeling good only about yourself or other people
- Being strong all the time
- Looking always outward and never inward

Take a minute to think about what constitutes psychological/emotional health. Would you include any of the above? Let's look at a different way of thinking.

Good psychological/emotional health includes the following:

- Ability to tolerate and experience all your feelings, even when they are intense and make you highly uncomfortable
- Ability to tolerate ambivalence and see more gray than black and white
- Willingness to look equally comfortably at your strengths and weaknesses
- Self-reflection
- Good balance of work and play
- Placing an equal value on independence and dependence
- Feeling generally positive and trusting of the world around you
- Valuing and craving genuine intimacy and also feeling comfortable with solitude
- Seeing both yourself and others as emotional resources
- Engaging in flexible, nonrigid thinking most of the time
- Valuing people over material things
- Asserting your needs and also respecting and valuing the needs of others
- Being open to new ways of thinking and doing but also maintaining strong convictions
- Finding meaning in living and being alive
- Looking for and finding people who treat you well
- Being able to laugh at yourself, especially at your mistakes
- Developing outlets for your creative abilities
- Being comfortable standing up for yourself when you are right and admitting when you are wrong

- Making mostly rational decisions that enhance your well-being
- Having the courage to take risks when they are to your long-term advantage and to refrain from risks when they're not
- Being willing to deal with your past, including childhood or adult trauma
- Expressing your needs directly
- Expecting that being an adult means you will not always be loved unconditionally
- Being accountable and taking responsibility for yourself
- Accepting that you are doing the best you can, even as you try to do better

The above list is not meant to be exhaustive, but it offers a window into qualities you can strive for to become more psychologically/emotionally sound. Please note that because you are human, *it is impossible to achieve or excel at every criterion.* Psychological/emotional health requires practice. None of us is in perfect psychological/emotional health because we're all recovering from childhood wounds of one kind or another. We are all perfectly imperfect!

It's important, too, to take into consideration how cultural values affect psychological/emotional health. For instance, western societies may value independence over teamwork; eastern ones may attach great importance to manners and saving face. Although it's necessary to be sensitive to cultural values, it's equally necessary to recognize these occasions when archaic values get in the way of psychological/emotional health.

One of the hallmarks of good psychological and emotional self-care is having a strong, unquestioned loyalty toward it. This means having an unequivocal desire to be good to yourself that isn't riddled with unconscious, conflicting feelings and doubts about whether you are worth it or not. Either you are or you aren't. Forget gray. Here's one area where black-and-white thinking is not only acceptable but imperative. Your decision about whether or not you're worth taking care of to the best of your ability rests at the heart of self-care—and, not surprisingly, it will either move you toward becoming a "normal" eater or be a barrier to it.

If you're uncertain about your deservedness and self-worth, you will surely sabotage your attempts at "normal" eating. So before throwing yourself into increased self-care efforts, take all the time you need to resolve this dilemma. Intrapsychic conflict impedes growth, change, and recovery and makes them more of a struggle. So make sure that you feel certain *you deserve to be good to you.*

If you meet many or most of the criteria for good psychological/emotional self-care, you're probably feeling pretty good about yourself in general. Continue to remain aware of what you're doing and thinking, be scrupulously honest with yourself even when it hurts, and be willing to go into unfamiliar territory and to change when your behavior or thinking isn't working for you. Whenever you find yourself being rigid, you're losing ground. Good emotional and psychological health care requires flexible reflection and action.

What constitutes good spiritual self-care?

In today's material world, spirituality is often sadly neglected. Eagerness for *doing* has eclipsed interest in simply *being* because when we try to listen to the still, small voice inside we are often visited by disquieting feelings and unsettling questions. If we can't answer them right away or if we feel pressure to come up with the "right" answer, we get scared and overwhelmed. So, rather than spending time in contemplation, we rush away from our confusion and uncertainty into the safety of known and familiar activities.

Spirituality has also become associated with organized religion and belief in God. Many people have given up on their spiritual selves because they were forced to worship at a church, synagogue, or mosque as a child or to attend a religious school that squelched their individualism, critical thinking skills, and uniqueness. Other people neglect their spiritual side because they believe that it's not crucial to their happiness or success, or they simply feel they don't have time for it. But spirituality is an internal feeling and you don't have to step inside a house of worship or believe in a supreme being to feel or nurture it.

Spirituality has to do with feeling connected to something larger than yourself and believing there is purpose to your life beyond meeting your personal needs. It has to do with revering the world and striving to make it a better place. Atheists and agnostics can be as spiritual as nuns, priests, rabbis, and ministers. Spirituality is the paradoxical ability to recognize your insignificance in the world as well as your grandness, your universality as well as your uniqueness, the fact that you and everything else in the world are sacred and special.

Good spiritual self-care includes but is certainly not limited to:

- Feeling connected to the earth, nature, and the humanity of everyone on the planet
- Having a sense of something larger than yourself, whether it is God or a higher power, or a community or purpose that lends meaning to your existence
- Looking for ways to feel the awesomeness of yourself, others, and the world
- Finding ways to give your unique gifts to the world
- Looking for opportunities to connect more profoundly to yourself, others, and the world around you
- Acting in moral, ethical, and rational ways
- Finding ways to deeply appreciate and honor people, places, and things
- Making emotional peace with illness, death, and the terrible things that happen on the planet, which means accepting and not denying that anything can happen to anyone at any time
- Coming to terms with your own mortality and the mortality of those you love
- Being open to new ways of looking at yourself in connection to the universe

One last word about spiritual self-care. Many people are not able to examine this part of their life until they've achieved a modicum of physical, mental, and psychological/emotional health. Imagine trying to discuss good and evil with a starving person: a good meal is needed to free them to think about other things. As Alcoholics Anonymous says, first things first. It's natural to try to build a comfortable physical, mental, and emotional foundation before embarking on less tangible endeavors. However, this is not a must. In fact, for many people, achieving spiritual centeredness is a precursor to physical, mental, and emotional soundness—if there's no meaning to life, why bother striving for any kind of health? People seek spirituality in many ways, so feel free to explore what works for you.

Will taking better care of myself help me become a "normal" eater?

I hope by now you accept that you've been doing your best to cope and take care of yourself even if you've been doing it by undereating or overeating. I hope you can also see that disordered eating has now become a problem in its own right. Not only does it not work *for* you, it works *against* you.

Taking better care of yourself is what's called a twofer: the price of one action buys you two great results. It will help you make enormous strides in becoming a "normal" eater, *and* it will provide you with the skills you need to live a more satisfying, enjoyable, healthy, successful life. The two go hand in hand. Once you stop repeatedly misinterpreting your self-care signals, mixing apples and oranges—pardon the pun—you'll stop confusing hunger with your emotional needs and start responding to each more appropriately. You'll end up turning to food abuse less often *and* to whatever rings your emotional chimes more often!

In fact, it isn't possible to have a serious restrictive eating problem or a severe compulsive/emotional eating problem *and* be taking good care of yourself physically and emotionally. If you're physically hungry and refuse yourself food, or if you're full and you keep eating, you're not taking care of your body. And if you're eating or restricting food instead of feeling your feelings, you're not taking care of yourself emotionally. These chronic patterns of disordered eating are antithetical to good self-care.

An exception in which good self-care means restriction is when your diet is constrained by a digestive disorder or bona fide food allergy. If you can view these constraints as nondeprivational, rational, healthy choices that you are making to maintain good health, there's no reason for them to impair your ability to lead a happy, productive life.

And remember, self-care does not mean never using food to lift your spirits. The major difference between "normal" and disordered eaters is the frequency with which they use food or food issues to take care of themselves and their reaction when they do. "Normal" eaters may occasionally take care of themselves by eating or not eating. They may skip a meal, make impulsive food choices, or overeat once in a while. They may be too busy to eat or ignore the rumblings in their stomach to comfort their child, clean the house before company arrives, meet with a client, or get to a movie on time. They may occasionally grab a candy bar at the checkout counter, delight in a slice of hot apple pie, or leave the table stuffed with holiday turkey. They find food tasty and delicious and sometimes it makes them feel better, but they don't depend on eating or not eating to take care of them.

Think of the relationship between self-care and disordered eating like this: whenever you eat or restrict food *based on your emotions*, you are preventing yourself from meeting an underlying emotional or physical need. You're ignoring and distracting yourself from a yearning inside that desires to be met in non-food-related ways. These needs will not simply go away, nor should they, because they represent an authentic, valuable, healthy part of you that needs to be attended to. Therefore, they must be addressed.

Here are some food-related examples that show how to honor yourself. By resisting the urge to weigh yourself when you're anxious and instead sitting with your feelings, you are building emotional muscle. When you take it slow but choose to finish the food on your plate because you're still hungry, you're responding to your body's need for fuel. When you pull your mind away from ruminating about overeating the previous night, you're disciplining yourself to live in the present. When you choose a dish of ice cream over a carrot without calculating the calories you're consuming, you are practicing giving yourself permission to experience pleasure. When you order a soufflé rather than your usual garden salad and eat without guilt, you're making a public statement about your right to enjoy food.

When you get home from work and hop on the treadmill for 30 minutes instead of gobbling down a bag of jelly beans, you are de-stressing your body. When you drag yourself off to bed instead of polishing off the moo shi shrimp you had for dinner, you are respecting your need for sleep. When you call a friend, go to a movie, write a letter to a family member, or take a walk instead of diving into the cookie jar when you're feeling blue, you're reminding yourself that you have the power to take care of your emotional needs. When you express your disappointment at someone who hurt you rather than skip your lunch with her, you are asserting that you have the right to honor your feelings.

Even as you begin to take better care of yourself and address your underlying emotional needs, your life will not get better instantly. Not eating emotionally, compulsively, or restrictively is only the first step. Doing whatever needs to be done to address your emotional needs is the second. Or you can reverse the order and start to address your emotional needs first, which will help you move toward "normal" eating. Both efforts are an essential part of good self-care, and the more you do one, the easier it will be to do the other.

If I believe I am a deserving person, will I take better care of myself?

Although many aspects of disordered eating are unconscious, both restrictive and compulsive/emotional eaters sometimes make conscious food decisions that are irrational. Nowhere is this kind of dysfunctional decision making more prevalent than around the issue of deservedness. Disordered eaters often suffer great confusion and doubt about whether they deserve to feel pleasure, and as a result they end up either denying themselves the foods they crave or overeating them.

For example, after a stressful day at work do you, as a compulsive eater, return home exhausted and zoom toward the kitchen? You might remind yourself, I know I probably shouldn't have a cookie, but I *deserve* a little treat to make up for my crummy day. Do you feel somewhat irritated, defensive, and self-righteous when you make this statement? Your actions say that you believe you merit compensation because you're stressed, and that compensation should be in the form of food. The motivation to feel better is admirable, but the belief about deservedness is twisted. Here's how.

There is absolutely no question that you are a deserving, worthwhile person. You are, I am, we all are. But when you base eating decisions on what you *deserve*, you're missing the point.

Yes, you *deserve* that cookie/cake/candy, etc. You deserve seconds, fifths, everything on the menu or in the bakery. If you defend your eating by saying that you deserve something to eat, you will never say no to food because you will always be deserving. Get it? The question isn't "Are you deserving?" but "Are you hungry?"

The fact that you have to *prove* you are deserving is a dead giveaway that you don't really believe it. Someone who feels truly deserving and is unconflicted about her self-worth won't think much about being deserving. It's a given. Telling yourself that you deserve to eat (or buy that pretty silk shirt you don't need or have your nails done at a place you can't afford) is merely a way of reassuring yourself. If you were absolutely certain you were a deserving person, why would you have to keep proving it over and over again, with food or anything else?

Restrictive eaters also have many doubts about being deserving. Perhaps you're prone to feeling that you're not entitled to the food in your refrigerator or to eating out at a restaurant, splurging on a fine meal to celebrate a special occasion, enjoying some of your old favorites at a family get-together, eating in front of others, or even pleasuring yourself with food. Unlike the compulsive eater who eats to prove that she *is* deserving, you *don't eat* as proof that you aren't. Consistently saying no to food is a way of reinforcing your negative thinking about yourself and denying that you are a worthy person. Eating and enjoying food is a way to nurture your feelings of self-worth until you feel genuinely deserving.

Neither attitude toward food demonstrates the truth: *you are a valuable, deserving person whether you eat or not.* Listen to yourself carefully to hear if you have a deservedness dilemma that gets played out in the food arena. Watch out for the phrases,

"I shouldn't . . . but I deserve" and "I should . . . but I don't deserve." They're both telltale indications that you are conflicted about your self-worth. If you're a compulsive eater, tell yourself that of course you *deserve* whatever it is you want to eat, but that the issue is hunger; the issue is craving. If you're a restrictive eater and want food, tell yourself that eating would be a good choice because you respect and honor your body's messages. Keep reminding yourself that if you deserve anything, it's to be healthy and feel safe and comfortable around food.

Disconnecting food from the issue of whether or not you deserve it frees you to focus on hunger, making satisfying choices, eating with awareness and enjoyment, and stopping when you're full or satisfied. Here's one area in which you can comfortably use the word always: you are *always* deserving. Work on keeping your feeling that you are deserving stable while allowing your feelings about food to fluctuate according to your bodily wants and needs.

9

DAUNTING EATING SITUATIONS

If I'm Gritting My Teeth, How Will I Eat?

I once asked a client who suffered terribly with emotional eating what her most daunting eating situation was—dinner at her parents' home, holidays, dining out with friends, or being alone in her apartment on a Saturday night. She shook her head after each mention. "What *is* it?" I asked. "Being awake," she answered, only half joking. Every day was a struggle for her whether she was at home or out, alone or with people, in a good or bad mood. She was drawn to food like a moth to flame.

For many overeaters and undereaters, every minute of the day holds enormous pressure to eat or not eat. Compulsive eaters are faced with the agony of saying no to food, restrictive eaters with saying yes. When you have a food obsession, whether you're drawn to or repelled by food, it rules your life;

any food-related occasion, even something as seemingly benign as grocery shopping, can induce panic and distress.

For many disordered eaters, a number of fairly universal situations either increase or diminish appetite. For some it's dining with family or friends. For others it's a party or facing the endless edibles of a buffet. Holiday festivities. Whether or not to grab a bite on the road. A dinner date. Eating at work. Lunch with a client. Some disordered eaters eat relatively normally in familiar settings, but become anxious outside their comfort zone.

Never fear. You can learn successful strategies for becoming more comfortable in any daunting eating situation. If a circumstance seems challenging, it's only because you haven't yet achieved the awareness or skill you need to eat "normally" in it. New learning includes putting in place sound, rational beliefs about eating in that situation, staying in touch with your feelings, and paying special attention to your behavior around food. As always, it helps if patience, practice, persistence, compassion, and curiosity are your constant companions.

What about eating in restaurants?

The rules of "normal" eating travel well and apply in eateries as well as your own kitchen. After all, restaurants are filled with "normal" eaters (as well as every other kind!), so dining out with ease and enjoyment must be possible. The idea, once again, is for you *consciously* to make decisions and behave in ways that "normal" eaters *instinctively* do. Keep at it, and eventually it will be relatively automatic for you too.

Eating out with comfort and pleasure is actually the end-point in a series of decisions you make before you even leave home. You don't magically arrive at a restaurant, do you, having been plucked out of your living room and plunked down at a table for four? No, you make a choice (alone or with others) about what time you want to eat and which restaurant you prefer. On rare occasions you may have no choice, such as when someone else is hosting a celebration. Other times, you generally have at least some input into the decisions.

It's up to you to make sure that you're eating at a restaurant you enjoy or at least think you'll enjoy. It's pretty easy to please yourself, but more of a challenge when you're dining with others. If you dislike Chinese food, or adore it but have already had it twice this week, say so. If you're dying for shrimp on the barbie, put your craving out there. If you've been dreaming of a particular restaurant all week, suggest it. If price, travel distance, atmosphere, or food preparation are going to ruin your meal, speak up. It's up to you to state your feelings and negotiate from there. You may not always get your way—"normal" eaters eat in places that aren't their first (or fifth) choice—but make a genuine attempt to take care of your needs, foodwise and otherwise. The point is to avoid ending up feeling like a victim in a situation in which you had a choice.

If you prefer to eat early or late, be proactive and mention a specific time or range of times when you anticipate being moderately hungry. Many disordered eaters just go along with whatever time someone suggests in fear of seeming selfish or causing a disagreement, or because they are used to taking care of others and not themselves. Whenever you agree to eat at a time that doesn't jibe with your appetite, you're doing yourself a serious disservice. Again, you might not always get your way, but there's a good chance you will. Moreover, you will have practiced honoring your body and asserting yourself.

Unfortunately, no matter how assertive you are, there are times when you will find yourself in an unappealing restaurant at a time that totally disrupts your meal schedule. You might arrive sick with hunger or with virtually no desire for food. You might be stuck staring at a menu that either leaves you cold or overwhelms you with too many exotic choices. You might wish you'd never come and that you were anywhere else besides at Cafe Wrong. In any of these cases, you might feel tempted to act out your feelings through food.

But remember, you have another option: to think how a "normal" eater would react. I can tell you that they definitely would not invest a great deal of emotional energy in this particular eating experience, and that they'd neither starve nor stuff themselves. They would simply mentally write off a lousy meal and move on. For you to be so cavalier about food might mean taking time to assess your mood, particularly if you're feeling resentful, disappointed, anxious, deprived, or angry. Once you've acknowledged your feelings, it's important to remind yourself that the meal will eventually come to an end. If you need space to come to terms with your feelings, by all means excuse yourself and find the bathroom, or phone home and leave a message for yourself about what's going on inside you. Return to the table only when you've achieved a more relaxed state of mind.

If you're overwhelmed with too many food choices on a menu, find the one thing you simply can't do without. Don't inquire what other people plan to eat, but focus on your own hunger level and cravings. If you're worried about being influenced by others' orders, put yours in first. If you don't want specific foods, ask the waiter not to bring them. If you really love a dish, order two portions of it! Don't watch your companions eating. Eating is neither comparative nor competitive; it's an absolutely unique experience.

Eating out without feeling judged is especially hard if you are underweight or overweight or feel self-conscious about your food issues. If you're overweight, you may feel that you're not entitled to order something high in calories. If you're underweight, you may feel that everyone wants and expects you to order something substantial, to put some meat on your bones. Nevertheless, your obligation is only to yourself. In fact, many of the judgments you believe others have about you may instead be your own thoughts projected onto them. If you're eating with people who really do make judgmental comments about your food intake, it's time to find healthier eating companions.

Sometimes you think you are hungry, but for whatever reason when you get to a restaurant, your appetite disappears. In that case, order appropriately. Go for a small portion of something you like, or order that special dish you've been dying for, eat a little, and take the rest home to eat when you can really enjoy it. Listen to your body and be flexible. Have a cup of soup or a dessert, a big glass of iced tea, or a rich latte. It's no crime that you misjudged your hunger, nothing to feel embarrassed or ashamed about. Even "normal" eaters misread their bodies.

Another problem for compulsive eaters is feeling full and satisfied, stopping eating, then continuing to mindlessly pick at their food just because it's still there. If this happens to you, call the waiter over as soon as you've finished and ask him or her to take away your food. Or ask your dinner companions to share what's left.

Eating in restaurants can be frightening for disordered eaters because they don't feel in charge of all the variables in the same way they can be at home. Restrictive eaters especially may feel so anxious eating out or in front of others that they wish they didn't have to eat at all. If you're a restrictive eater who has difficulty eating out, be kind and patient with yourself. Know that the experience may be difficult and even painful, but that it will grow easier as you practice the rules of "normal" eating. Remind yourself that eating out is intended to be pleasurable, and let the rules give you the guidance you need to feel right with food no matter where you're eating.

Is it possible to eat "normally" with my family of origin?

Yes, it's possible to eat "normally" with family, but it can also be enormously challenging and require radical shifts in thinking, feeling, and behaving, along with a good deal of practice. If you're thinking you can read this section and then head off for a Sunday dinner of "normal" eating with your folks, forget it. While I do believe that if you put your mind to it, you can learn to eat "normally" in most, if not all, settings, it's crucial that you understand the power of your family of origin to trigger destructive eating. Families can set off your internal firecrackers and make every dining experience the Fourth of July. Prepare yourself, and think of the family dinner table as a high combustion area!

There are many reasons that family members may trigger undereating or overeating, and nearly all of them lurk beneath the surface of consciousness. For example, intrapsychic conflicts or tensions within each person often masquerade as interpersonal conflicts—tensions between people—so that two people who have conflicting feelings on a subject end up arguing about it instead of owning that they both have mixed feelings. The more readily you recognize the underlying *dine-amics* going on within your family, the better armed you will be to avoid reacting to them. Strive to understand what's being played out, and you will have won half the battle.

A major reason that food sets off our firecrackers is the relationship it plays between mother and child. Remember that your mother's first major task was to feed you in utero, then by breast or bottle, and that if she failed in this responsibility, you would have died. This dynamic created a powerful, special, intense bond that may still exist for you both. You grew inside her body, you were a part of her, and she may forget that you have been living outside her womb for 18, 33, or 62 years.

From your side of the table, of course, everything looks completely different. Precisely because you were so helpless and dependent on her—and who among us enjoys being dependent and helpless?—you may have spent much of your life struggling to prove that you are now independent. Primary in this struggle is the resolve you may now feel about managing your own food needs—proof positive to yourself, Mom, and the world that you are independent of her. On the other hand, if you were unable to adequately depend on your mother, you may have an unacknowledged wish to crawl right back inside her. Or, like so many of us, you may have conflicting feelings about dependence and independence.

Of course, not every mother and father is obsessed with nourishing their progeny, nor is every child on a crusade to feed herself. However, an inherent potential for conflict exists in the parent-child relationship when it comes to food. If your mother or father is still pushing food on you, begging or scolding you to eat or not eat, telling you what foods are good and bad for you, giving unsolicited culinary advice, dropping off little goodies on your doorstep, or in any other way intruding into your food world, try to understand that they are acting like, well, a parent. I'm not justifying their actions, only explaining that their actions are about *their* needs (for example, to feel needed by you, to not worry about you, to be perceived as a caring parent). They are not a reflection of your ability to care for yourself. Their behavior may have nothing to do with your capabilities at all. Soon we'll get to strategies for dealing with Mom and Dad, but for now let's just acknowledge the underlying biology and tremendous complexity of these issues.

Another reason it may be upsetting to eat with family is embedded in the memories of past family meals. If they were less than harmonious, if there were outbursts of yelling, blaming, flinging back chairs, and members storming off in a huff, you may still come to the family table quaking inside and expecting a violent row. If meals were silent, uptight affairs where the only words spoken were requests to pass around food, you may still harbor fears about opening your mouth for anything. If your parents argued throughout every meal and you were stuck in your chair tense and helpless, feeling like a monkey in the middle, you may feel trapped and panicky as you sit with them now. If your parents didn't prepare food adequately or feed you enough as a child, you may come to their table feeling angry at their neglect.

If your parents have or had eating or weight problems, their anxiety may permeate your experience of eating with them. A parent may worry about you becoming like them, eating too much, too little, or the "wrong" foods. If Mom or Dad is on a constant diet, they may feel threatened that you're eating something they don't allow themselves. Your attempts to eat less—or more—in your struggle to eat "normally" may stir up feelings of discomfort about their own dysfunctional eating habits, and they may be jealous and angry that you are accomplishing something they cannot. Your parents' negative attitude about your eating doesn't mean you are doing something wrong; in fact, it may mean that you are doing something right!

Although it's difficult not to take personally comments your relatives make about your eating, body, or weight, it helps to recognize that they may not have the foggiest idea that they're doing anything wrong. As a youngster, you may have looked up to them as all-powerful and all-knowing, but now that you've grown up, it's important to recognize that the words that come out of their mouths are more about *them* than about *you*. At the least, they certainly know far less about what your body wants than you do.

So many echoes from past meals may haunt today's family dinner table that you feel as if you're caught in a time warp. You are. It's so easy for family members to slip into old roles that it's more likely to happen than not. But you won't be thrown off course if you remain conscious of family dynamics and react as an adult, not as if you're still a child. You may need to educate your family about your new way of eating and thinking about food and your body. In fact, you may need to keep educating them over and over because eating "normally" may be a new, alien, suspicious, or dangerous concept to them. Or, you may have to give up on education, allow them to remain "ignorant," and simply continue to do what you have to do to get healthy.

Unconscious, unhealthy (but totally understandable!) reactions to eating with family come from years of being triggered. Before you realize it, all your firecrackers are blasting at once: you've been hurt, you feel vulnerable, and in your pain all you want to do is strike back. Unconscious reactions do nothing to move a situation toward resolution, however; in fact, the opposite is true and your knee-jerk response not only wounds others, but leaves you feeling ashamed and sometimes even more vulnerable. You may then be tempted to turn to food or obsessing about eating and weight issues to manage these feelings.

The following are dysfunctional, most-often unconscious reactions to problems that arise from eating with family:

- Overeating
- Undereating
- Refusing to eat
- Arguing about food
- Arguing about what you want or don't want to put into your body
- Putting down anyone who is dieting
- Making unsatisfying food choices
- Letting your feelings dictate your food choices and how much or how little you eat
- Disconnecting from your body
- Disconnecting from your feelings
- Storming away from the table
- Giving your family the silent treatment
- Criticizing the way family members are eating or what they weigh
- Blaming family members for making you eat more or less than you intended
- Suffering in silence and viewing yourself as a victim of a dysfunctional family
- Playing the martyr and rejecting food

- Making excuses for relatives who try to control your eating because "they mean well"
- Feeling trapped at the table even if family members become abusive or violent
- Eating whatever is put on your plate so your family will love you
- Punishing someone by not eating food that was made specially for you and that you would normally enjoy
- Defending what you are eating or not eating
- Trying futilely to explain "normal" eating to family members who are unable to take in what you have to say

Conscious, healthy responses, on the other hand, come from a peaceful, rational, goal-oriented place inside you. Responding with awareness and positive intent make all the difference. Yes, you may be hurt, but it's neither appropriate nor effective to "fight back." Believe me, I am hardly suggesting that you be passive or go along with your family's dysfunction, around eating or anything else. Far from it. It takes a tremendous amount of work to *think rationally* when people around you are acting irrationally. But this is exactly what you need to do to manage your feelings and behave in a healthy manner, and you can achieve this goal with heightened awareness and practice. Developing healthy reactions to family members concerning food and weight issues will not only help you become a "normal" eater, but will improve your relationships with them and make you feel better about yourself.

Whether you're working on feeling comfortable with eating or not eating around your family, there's work to do on two fronts: changing yourself and changing your relationships. Changing yourself means reaching inside yourself for a rational, healthy response that you can be proud of rather than reacting to feeling wounded. Changing your relationships means trying to improve communication between you and a family member, such as gently confronting those who try to force-feed you as if you were an infant, or firmly standing up for yourself when your family gangs up on you to eat or not eat.

Putting words in your mouth for family situations

Although there's no one-size-fits-all response to family members who try to thwart your efforts to become a "normal" eater, here are a few responses that you can use as is or tweak to fit your particular situation. Remember, these suggestions are for changing the relationship. Most of the time, you can only change you. Sometimes, perhaps often, you will have nothing to say because you're too busy focusing your energies inside yourself and doing whatever you know is right for you!

Refusing Food That Is Offered or Served to You

- Thanks, I know you made it specially for me, but I'm not hungry right now.
- I'd like to take it home and eat it later when I'll really enjoy it.
- If I ate it now, it would be a waste because I'm too full to enjoy it.
- I appreciate your making this for me and it's really hard for me to say no, but I need to.
- Please don't think my refusal means I don't value all the work you put into making these.

- I'm going to have one bite now and save the rest for later.
- Thanks for understanding, but I can't eat that right now.

Responding to Comments About How Little You Are Eating

- I know you worry about me, but I'm an adult and you no longer need to.
- Believe me, I do eat when I'm hungry.
- It makes me upset when you focus on my eating.
- I'm not comfortable when you push me to eat, so I'd appreciate it if you wouldn't.
- I'm trying to listen to my body, and right now it's had enough.
- I'm not hungry right now, but maybe later on I will be.
- Like any "normal" eater, sometimes I'm hungry and sometimes I'm not.
- I prefer to talk about something other than food.
- My recovery depends on honoring the messages my body gives me about when and what to eat. You can really help by supporting me in that.

Responding to Comments About How Much You Are Eating

- I know you worry about me, but I'm an adult and you no longer need to.
- I'm really hungry right now.
- I'm trying to listen to when my body tells me I've had enough.
- When I'm no longer hungry, I'll stop eating.

- Sometimes I do overeat, and I'm working on doing it less.
- I'm uncomfortable when you focus on what I eat.
- I know you mean well, but your comments about my eating only upset me, and when I'm upset I sometimes eat more.

Responding to Comments About Your Weight (Gain or Loss)

- I'm uncomfortable when you make comments about my weight gain/loss.
- I know you mean well, but I'd prefer it if you didn't comment on my weight, and I'll be glad to explain why.
- I'm pretty touchy about my weight, and hearing comments about it makes me upset.
- Yes, I have lost/gained weight, but I'd rather it not be a focus of discussion.
- I would be so much happier if you didn't bring up my weight.
- I'm self-conscious about my weight gain/loss, so please let's not talk about it.
- Yes, I do struggle with my weight, and I'm getting help with the problem.

Commenting When Table Talk Is All About Food or Dieting

- Anyone seen any good movies lately or read any interesting books?
- Does anyone else find it hard to enjoy eating when all we're talking about is food?
- I'd love to hear about that low-fat recipe, but let's wait till after dinner.

- Let's see how long we can go without talking about food or dieting.
- I'm finding it hard to focus on enjoying my food with all this talk about fat grams and calories.
- I'd rather focus on what I am eating than what I'm not.

It's important to try to talk to your family members about how you feel with them around food, but not everyone is going to understand or even want to hear you out. If you sense genuine interest in what you have to say, by all means explain why and how you're working on becoming a "normal" eater. But if you sense disinterest or antagonism, let the subject go. Remember that it took *you* a while to be ready for the concept of eating consciously. Moreover, many dieters and compulsive eaters will be so threatened by what you have to say that they feel they have to turn you off.

Your job is not to convince your entire family that "normal" eating is right for you. Your job is only to convince yourself and then make your own choices.

When I'm with friends or a lover, how can I keep focused on the rules of "normal" eating?

Social eating situations often make it difficult to stay grounded in your body and aware of what it wants. Let's look at some reasons why eating with friends or a lover can throw you off course. One is that conversation is a distraction from eating mindfully. Ideally, you could do both—listen, ask questions, tell funny stories, contribute your share to the conversation *and* eat. This is what "normal" eaters do automatically, the same way that you talk on the phone while putting away the groceries or sing along with your favorite CD while backing into a parking space. When you were learning to drive, however, I'll bet that all your brain cells were focused exclusively on that effort. You may need that same narrowed concentration to learn to eat "normally."

Are you someone who completely loses herself in conversation and forgets what's going into your mouth? Then you might do well to minimize social eating until you're able to stay connected to your body *and* enjoy your mealtime companionship. Check your readiness by talking on the phone while you're eating to see if you can maintain a dual focus. If you can, try going for a cup of tea or coffee or a light lunch with one person, and notice whether you're able to concentrate on the conversation *and* your food. When you're ready, try eating with two or three people. In general, if you're effective at multitasking, you may have an easier time with social eating than if you easily get distracted or overwhelmed. In that case, eating with friends or a lover may be a real challenge. You may need a considerable amount of practice in eating mindfully by yourself before you venture out into social eating situations.

Eating with friends or a lover may also be difficult because you feel self-conscious. Reframing your beliefs about being judged can go a long way toward relaxing you, as can maintaining body awareness. And, if someone does comment on your eating, this presents an excellent opportunity to change the relationship by talking about your feelings either on the spot or after the meal. Remember, judgmental remarks may be an indicator that *others* have a hidden eating problem. If someone continues to make remarks that cause you discomfort after you've told them so, it may be time to reevaluate the relationship. Alternatively, once you've become more of a "normal" eater, other people's comments may not bother you. "Normal" eaters may or may not find intrusive comments annoying, but they certainly don't act out with food when they hear them.

Social eating can be problematic when emotions run high and threaten to overwhelm you. If you and a lover quarrel during a meal, your energies are likely to go toward protecting your vulnerability and not toward eating "normally." And when you're upset, you may feel a strong urge to fall back into unsatisfying food choices and ignore your hunger and satiation signals. If you're arguing with a friend or lover during a meal, either stop the row or stop eating; one of the activities has to go. If you're dining out, ask the waiter for a doggie bag; if you're at home, take your disagreement into another room and finish it away from the table.

Dining with others can be troublesome if table talk centers around food or dieting. Unfortunately, the dos and don't's of eating have become common conversational fare these days. Nothing ruins enjoyment faster than some well-intended person pointing out the number of calories or fat grams in the sandwich you're about to bite into. Talk of food plans, body fat calibrations, nutrition, or weigh-ins may also stir up uneasy feelings.

Sadly, when you begin to follow a path toward "normal" eating, you may find yourself traveling alone. With luck, you can get one or two friends to take the journey with you. If not, you may feel a widening breach between yourself and your diet or binge companions. They may not understand why you no longer want to hear about their experiences with food, and they may feel rejected by you. You, on the other hand, may want to avoid all talk of dieting because of the attraction it still holds for you.

As with family, it's worth a try to explain the theory behind "normal" eating to friends and lovers. Work on understanding where their fears and doubts lie and, if you can, address them. Be patient and encourage them to ask questions. Don't feel you have to be the authority on the subject. Lend them a book or an article, or direct them to an anti-diet website. Suggest a workshop you've taken. Tell them you know the idea might seem revolutionary and that you're available to talk more about "normal" eating whenever they like.

A discussion about eating with friends would not be complete without addressing the issues of self-sabotage and friendly fire. Sometimes, out of fear of changing too quickly and to slow ourselves down, we sabotage our progress, most often unconsciously. If someone else is trying to sabotage your progress, it's likely that they feel threatened (probably also unconsciously) by the changes you're making and are trying to get you to revert to your old, familiar behavior. If a friend or lover has an eating or weight problem, relationship insecurities, or emotional issues, he or she might be frightened by your new approach to food. When you get your life together, will you still want this person in it? If you're able to succeed at becoming a "normal" eater, does that mean they're a failure? If you continue changing, will the two of you have anything in common? They may harbor mixed feelings: wanting you to achieve your eating goals and, at the same time, dreading your triumphs—so that sometimes you feel they're on your side and sometimes you don't.

Signs that a friend or lover is trying to sabotage your eating success include:

- Telling you that you'll never become a "normal" eater
- Attacking the concept of "normal" eating

- Giving you diet books to read
- Attempting to get you to binge with them or tempting you with foods you're trying to avoid
- Teasing you about how much or little you're eating
- Continuing behaviors you have asked them to stop (such as commenting on what you are eating or not eating, or on whether you've gained or lost weight)
- Making sarcastic comments about your progress
- Distancing themselves from you in subtle ways
- Telling you they liked you better before you started to change
- Insisting that you were more fun to be with when you were dieting or bingeing

Allowing lovers or friends to sabotage your recovery from disordered eating is simply another way of sabotaging yourself and acting like a victim. Self-sabotage may indicate that you're ambivalent about change, which is perfectly natural and consistent with the recovery process. Most of us are conflicted about major change because it involves not only gain, but loss. However, even if you do have mixed feelings, sabotaging yourself is not an effective way of managing them. Instead, try to appreciate and understand your mishmashed—even polarized—emotions. Take the pressure off yourself to change overnight, and give yourself permission to slow down.

You are responsible only for *your* thoughts, feelings, and actions. You cannot predict how becoming a "normal" eater will affect your friendships or relationship with a partner. Personal transformation involves leaving friends and lovers who cannot relate to or support the new, healthy you. Sad as it is at the time, the loss of companions can present a wonderful opportunity to bring new people into your life, especially if they are healthy and on your wavelength. *If you want to succeed, becoming a "normal" eater may need to be the most important goal in your life*—more important than your wife, husband, parents, kids, job, friends, clients, or colleagues.

Is there really a way to eat "normally" at parties, potlucks, and buffets?

If "normal" eaters manage to feel comfortable eating at large social gatherings, there must be a way, right? The only reason you doubt the possibility is because of your current or former view that eating is a big, scary deal. Think of it this way, if you were injured in a nasty car wreck in your youth, you might be afraid of driving or even riding in a car. But if your childhood didn't include an auto accident, you'd feel reasonably OK about being a passenger or learning to drive.

Similarly, someone who hasn't suffered from disordered eating has no cause to feel uneasy about any kind of food event because they know they can depend on their body to tell them what and how much to comfortably eat. You, on the other hand, may assume you won't have a clue and, therefore, view buffets, catered affairs, and holiday parties as frightening occasions.

Attending a feast or any large- or medium-sized social gathering where the emphasis is on food—or even an intimate soiree with a wider variety of foods than you're used to—may feel like asking someone who can't swim to dive in head first and swim the English Channel. Fearing eating or overeating, you might make excuses and chronically avoid such gatherings. You might go and then end up eating everything in sight, or attend but strictly will yourself to eat nothing no matter how hungry you are.

One of the main reasons you have trouble at feasts is that you expect to. A "normal" eater receives an invitation to a black-tie charity banquet and starts digging out the tux or grandmother's pearls. If you're a compulsive undereater, you hear the word banquet and immediately tense up, thinking how hard it's going to be to pass up all that delicious food. You're thinking, *I won't eat all day, so I won't gain weight if I eat too much at the banquet. I'll exercise longer, and then I'll be able to enjoy myself. I'll drink a lot of water and stay away from the food so it won't tempt me. I'll eat nothing but foods that are nonfattening.* If you're a compulsive overeater, the idea of attending a banquet will start you obsessing about what "forbidden" foods you might run into. You're thinking, *with all those great foods, I know I'll overeat. I'll never be able to stay away from the dessert table. It's a party, so it's OK if I eat till I'm sick because everyone does.*

You may not realize that this anxiety-provoking chatter is programming your future behavior, particularly if they are supported by beliefs about your inability to feel comfortable around food. To act rationally and in your own best interests at feasts, you have to first *think rationally*. It's rational to believe that:

- The situation will be challenging
- You will try your best to make healthy choices
- You might make mistakes by eating too much or too little
- You can use whatever happens to understand yourself better and make better decisions next time

Several factors may make feasts difficult: the sheer quantity of food, the large variety of "forbidden" foods, the focus on cocktail chatter and small talk which may not be your strong suit, and the atmosphere of forced gaiety and elevated mood which you might not share. Not only are you faced with enormous food quantities, but it's all those goodies you've been denying yourself for weeks, months, or even years. And instead of approaching them in a relaxed, calm, composed state, you are confronting them when you feel pressure to put on your best social self.

Nevertheless, by sticking to the rules of "normal" eating—and learning a few other simple techniques—you can exchange your fear of food for an accepting attitude of delight in coming face to face with a luscious variety of foods. The first change is to reframe all your irrational beliefs about feasts, which have to do with good and forbidden or bad foods, weight gain, deprivation, your need or inability to control yourself around food, and caring what others think about your eating or not eating. Make a list of what you think "normal" eaters believe about feasts and read it over until the beliefs sound like something you might think. Every time an irrational, disordered eating belief about feasts flits across your mental screen, gently replace it with a rational "normal" eating one.

Once your beliefs about feasts are healthy and rational, you should notice a change in your feelings. No longer will you feel uptight and frightened; instead, you will begin feeling capable and up to the experience of being around all sorts of delectable foods. If you lose that feeling, you may realize you have allowed an irrational fear to slip back into its old slot. Pay lots of attention to your feelings. If you start to feel anxious about the food ahead of you, soothe yourself to gently reduce your anxiety.

Before the feast, visualize yourself eating with awareness, with the pleasure and delight that only true trust in and connection with your body can bring. Do this mental exercise on the train or bus, in the car at red lights, before going to sleep, when you awake, during TV commercials, while you're brushing your teeth, in boring meetings, as you're washing the dishes, in the checkout line in the supermarket. By envisioning yourself eating with awareness and pleasure and trusting your body, you're laying the neurological groundwork for future behavior. And, don't forget the best part: imagining how proud you'll feel after the feast, when you've eaten with mindfulness and enjoyment. The taste of success is the sweetest treat of all!

Remind yourself what the purpose of the feast is: to celebrate a holiday, birthday, wedding, anniversary, bat or bar mitzvah, promotion, or other occasion. If you know who will be there, think ahead of people you want to catch up with. If you won't know any or many people, acknowledge that you may feel nervous and lonely. When you arrive, assess your hunger level. It's good to be a little hungry—just hungry enough to eat—but it's OK if you're not. Trust your body to be there for you and tell you exactly what it wants and doesn't want.

If your hunger level tells you it's time to eat and there's a buffet, first check out all the food so you will be prepared to make informed, satisfying choices. Take your time. These are important decisions your body is making. Don't let anyone rush you, even if you're holding up the line or have to let people skip ahead of you.

Pretend you're shopping, looking for that perfect something, and you won't settle for anything less. Pick the top three to five foods you'd like to try and mindfully eat a little bit of each. Then ask yourself if you're still hungry. If not, wait a while. Talk to people, make a trip to the bathroom, or wander around the room observing others. Monitor your mood. If you are still hungry, sample a couple of other foods or take small helpings of seconds from your top favorites. Be grateful that you don't have to try everything because you'd be painfully full. Feel proud that you have the ability to be selective.

If you tend to overeat, tell yourself that you *could* try everything but you don't want to, that you *could* eat more, but you'd prefer not to feel stuffed. Focus on what you *are* eating, not the foods you haven't chosen. Remind yourself that there will be another time, at another feast, when you are hungry again.

If you tend to deny yourself the foods you want, tell yourself that it's OK to eat foods you love, that you *could* say no to anything and everything, but that you'd prefer to eat "normally" and sample some of the foods you enjoy. Focus on the foods your body craves, not the calorie calculator in your head. Remind yourself that you are entitled to eat and by making satisfying food choices, you are becoming a healthier person.

The biggest mistake people make at feasts is trying a little bit of everything. You could probably get away with that if you were a sumo wrestler, but it won't work for an average-sized person. Remember, feasts are not an all-or-nothing affair. You can make choices about the kinds of and quantities of foods you want to eat. Listen to what your body says about hunger, possible selections, enjoyment, and satisfaction. As soon as you're full or satisfied and have stopped eating, get rid of your plate, move away from the food table, and turn those cheerleaders inside your head up to full volume. You did it! You ate when you were hungry, made satisfying choices, ate with awareness and enjoyment, and stopped at satiation. Hurray for you!

If you're truly not hungry at a feast but have the urge to continue eating anyway, notice the feeling and let it pass. Return to lavishly praising yourself for eating "normally," and find someone to talk to or somewhere to go. If you aren't having a good time, either do something to improve your mood or give yourself permission to leave. One caution. If you're prone to self-sabotage or have difficulty tolerating positive feelings about yourself, you might arrive home after a sterling success with "normal" eating and head right for the refrigerator to undo those proud emotions. Or ignore your hunger the next time it says to eat. Instead, try to understand why it's so difficult to tolerate feeling good about yourself. Let the inclination to undo your achievement pass and if you think you're about to give in, find something to do, leave the house, take a shower, write in your journal, call a friend, or go to sleep. If you do end up eating or starving yourself, you can still drag out those cheerleaders, though. Remind yourself that you did a bang-up job at the feast, and next time you'll do even better in the aftermath.

Please don't forget that "normal" eaters overindulge at times, especially at feasts! So, if you do eat beyond the point of fullness or satisfaction, just accept the fact as a "normal" eater would and don't eat again until you're hungry. Wait an hour, an afternoon, or until the next day. If you have a tendency to punish yourself for overeating by *not* eating the next time you're hungry, remind yourself that this is unhealthy and hurtful behavior, and that you're entitled to respond to your body's appetite cues even though you recently disregarded them. Remember that you're learning to be less hard on yourself, and that although you can't undo what you did, you can make a healthy choice right now.

Trust your body to regulate what you need even when your mind can't. You can override anxiety by applying compassion and rational thinking. Ask yourself what a "normal" eater would do in your situation, then do it!

10

BODY ACCEPTANCE

I Get It—Keep the Body, Change the Attitude!

Now that you've arrived at the final chapter of this book, your head may be spinning. You may be in a panic, as many of my students are in the last session of my eating workshops—*Oh, no, I didn't learn everything I need to become a "normal" eater! This is the biggest challenge I've ever had in my life, and I'm not sure I can do it!* The ideas I've proposed may seem so radical and alien, so unlike you that you can't imagine yourself *ever* eating normally.

However, if you've gotten all the way to the last chapter of this book, it's obvious that being a disordered eater is very troubling to you and that you're seriously looking for a way to feel more at ease around food. If you're still reading, it means that you want to think and behave differently. That doesn't mean you don't have fears and questions about the future;

you probably do have mixed feelings, which is normal and healthy.

One of your biggest fears may be not about whether you can learn to eat "normally" but about what will happen to your body if you start feeding it the foods it wants. Large or small, you might be terrified of putting on weight, especially after you've spent a lifetime under the pressure to be thin. If you're fat, you might fear that becoming a "normal" eater could mean you'll grow even larger. If you're thin, you may have convinced yourself that it's OK to have an eating problem if it keeps your weight down.

Let's reiterate the main point of this book: to comfort and defeat your fears, you'll need to develop a new, rational, healthy belief system about your weight. In fact, changing your attitudes toward food might seem like a piece of cake compared to the idea of accepting your body, whatever its shape or size. You might think that you could eventually learn to become a "normal" eater, while you can't imagine ever accepting and loving your body as it is.

This chapter will help you explore body and weight beliefs so that you can decide how to change your thinking to accommodate your body, rather than how to change your body to accommodate your thinking!

How can I learn to be more accepting of my body and everyone else's?

It's nearly impossible to live in today's culture and not be prejudiced against fat. With the media insisting that thin equals success and diet plans equating slenderness with health and fitness, you may not even realize the ways in which you're being bombarded on a daily basis with pro-thin, anti-fat messages. Our society's obsession with carbs and calories makes slim and trim seem like the only worthwhile goal in life, especially for women. While even "normal" eaters and people of average weight may harbor judgmental feelings about fat, the issue is especially troublesome for disordered eaters. Because you don't trust your body and tend to define your value by its size, you're particularly sensitive and susceptible to negative messages about fat. And because you're not very accepting of your own body, you're probably judgmental about everyone else's.

Like every other transformation, moving from rejecting to accepting your body is a process that takes time and a willingness to risk experiencing yourself in new and unfamiliar ways. Even though you may be unhappy about being judgmental about your body, these feelings of dissatisfaction, disgust, or disappointment have become familiar and predictable. Replacing them with positive feelings is unsettling and scary. In fact, hatred for your body can feel so normal and natural that you can't envision feeling any other way.

There are two lines of thinking about what's wrong with fat: the first is that it's unhealthy. However, the fact is that weight is *not* the sole determinant of good or poor health or life expectancy. You can be fit *and* fat, if you reduce your health risks by exercising and making healthy lifestyle choices. If your concern about being fat or thin is health-related, then there are actions you can take to get and stay healthy while you're working toward finding a natural weight for your body through "normal" eating.

The other train of thought about fat is that it's unattractive and a person who has too much of it is bad. This judgment has nothing to do with health and everything to do with your self-perception and the influence of external forces. Rejecting fat because it's supposedly unattractive is, in plain English, stinkin' thinkin'. These perceptions are opinion, not fact—they are arbitrary, nonsensical, irrational smoke and mirrors. A huff and a puff will blow their house down.

One way to begin the shift away from body rejection is to wonder why you dislike fat so intensely. Are you using your negative feelings as a motivator, convinced that if only you hate your fat enough, you'll lose weight or never gain a pound? Do you fear that if you accept your body, you'll grow fat or fatter? Perhaps you believe that fat is bad because that's what everyone else thinks. It's certainly what our media and cultural messages constantly convey, both overtly and covertly.

Maybe you put your energy into judging your body because it's more comfortable than focusing on other unsatisfying aspects of yourself or your life—your lack of ambition, parenting problems, feeling trapped in a job or lifestyle that brings you little pleasure, being without a partner or staying with one you're unhappy with, growing up and away from your parents, or growing old. Keeping the spotlight on your body helps you avoid acknowledging other problems that are lurking in the shadows. Ask yourself: If I stop focusing on my body—fat or thin—what else about my life would upset me?

Along with understanding what you get out of hating fat and judging your body, it's necessary to review your beliefs to uncover irrational, unhealthy cognitions. If you believe that fat is ugly, what's your evidence? What's so inherently awful about fat? Nothing. Fat is just a bunch of cells. Views of fat and thin are culture-specific and time-bound. Rather than believing that fat is ugly, why not believe it's beautiful, or feel neutral about it? Why not focus on health rather than weight? Remember, you have a choice about what to believe about fat, thin, your body, and everything else.

Once you've identified your irrational beliefs about weight and size, go through and reframe each of them to make them rational and healthy. Work on developing a belief system about fat and your body that sounds something like this:

- Fat is neither bad nor good. It's merely extra cells.
- Beauty comes in all sizes—fat, thin, and in-between.
- I can decide how I feel about fat.
- I can believe whatever I want about my body.
- Loving my body is better than hating it; accepting it is better than rejecting it.
- My body is meant to function, not be judged.
- Focusing on disliking my body makes me avoid other issues in my life that need attention.
- Being too thin can be unhealthier than being fat.
- I can love and accept my body no matter what its size and shape.
- I can be both fat and fit.
- Only I can decide what I think about fat and thin.
- Being too thin is a dangerous obsession that has no appeal to me.
- There's nothing wrong with me or anyone else because of being fat.
- Being fat or thin does not make me good or bad, worthwhile or worthless.
- Being thin is not better than being fat.

- Putting on weight is not necessarily a bad thing.
- I can change my thinking about fat and thin.

In an intensely fat-phobic and fat-loathing society, it takes tons of courage and self-confidence to stand up and say that fat is neither bad nor ugly, it simply *is*. It's especially hard to challenge the cultural norm if you *are* fat. But the fact is that you either buy into the fat-is-bad myth, or you don't. And if you don't, it's vital that you speak up and fight the damage that fat phobia is doing to you and everyone else, regardless of their size.

Fat phobia can cause large-bodied people to feel terrible about themselves to the extent that their life purpose becomes focused on losing weight instead of improving their health, calling a truce with food, and making an important contribution to the world. It drives some people to dangerous ultrathinness in order to feel acceptable and accepted, loved and lovable. The sad fact is that many underweight people don't even realize that they are driven by fat phobia. Remember, size is only part of who you are—one aspect, not the whole. It's merely one among hundreds of physical and nonphysical traits that make you unique (for example, traits such as tall, short, smart, creative, musical, empathic, spirited, witty, profound, understanding, soft-spoken, muscular, surefooted, brilliant, zany, efficient, generous, nimble, well organized, caring, trustworthy, practical, mechanical, and artistic).

If you judge other people by their weight, you probably find it hard not to judge yourself. Why are you so judgmental? Where do these damaging ideas come from? Why would it occur to you to think less of someone because of their shape or size? Why would you think less of yourself? Because you are judgmental, do you assume that others are too?

Ask yourself whether you're willing to live by a set of arbitrary ideals about what people, especially women, should and should not look like. Will you continue to support ridiculous standards that are nearly impossible to achieve and are detrimental to a sound mind and healthy body? Moreover, whether you're big or small, buying into the "Thin is better than fat" myth practically ensures that you'll always be at war with food. To make peace, you need to let eating "normally" determine what you will weigh, rather than allowing the desire to be a certain weight determine your food intake.

Stop yourself when you see that you're caught up in judging your body or someone else's. Examine what feels good about being critical and what feels bad about it. You may decide that you really don't want to hate anything or anyone because it's not a worthwhile emotion. Or you may realize that you are substituting the fear of fat for another feeling such as sadness or disappointment. Is it easier to dislike your body than your disordered eating? Is it more comfortable and familiar to think negatively about your body than to focus on other things you don't like about yourself or your other circumstances?

Changing your beliefs about fat, thin, weight, body shape, and size will be a slow, arduous process. Most of your negative feelings about your body stem from unconscious beliefs that you'll have to dig deep to uncover. You even may be surprised at how much animus you feel about fat, and the intensity of the feeling may shame or frighten you. If so, acknowledge that you feel as you do and move on to reframing your beliefs. Work on your beliefs about body shape, size, and weight until you have made them conscious and rational. If you believe that right now you cannot possibly love your body, work on developing a belief that's at least more neutral. The key is to accept that this is the body you have right now, that it has far more value than its appearance, and that you're working to make it healthier.

Accepting your body will go a long way toward helping you become a "normal" eater. If you don't value your body, why bother attending to what it has to say about hunger, eating pleasure, satisfaction, and fullness? If you don't value your body, why listen to its cravings and nourish it with healthy food? The truth is, you cannot hate your body and love yourself.

Is it a good idea for me to weigh myself regularly?

I can't stress strongly enough that by addressing your eating problems, your weight will take care of itself. After all, how could a scale possibly tell you how hungry or full you are, or whether you'd rather have a slice of pie or a slice of pineapple? If you're eating "normally," then your weight will go up or down to arrive at the most healthy point for your body. Your weight may even stay the same, except that now, instead of struggling with a dysfunctional relationship with food, you'll be more in harmony with your appetite because you'll be following the rules of "normal" eating.

That said, there are experts on both sides of the weigh-in debate. Some anti-diet advocates maintain that weekly, monthly, or occasional weight checks are OK to help you trust your body as you try out new eating and lifestyle habits. Other authorities insist that you'll never become a "normal" eater unless you throw your scale out the window immediately, because focusing on weight is one of the major causes of eating problems. I prefer not to take sides because, once again, only *you* know what will work best. So take a leap of faith and trust that by adhering to the rules of "normal" eating, you'll settle into a weight that's right for you.

Bear in mind the following questions when you're making decisions about weighing yourself (I use the plural *decisions* to remind you that you can change your mind about weighing yourself any time). Consider why you feel the need to weigh yourself. Are you addicted to the process? Do you weigh yourself as a way of controlling your food intake? To see what you can or cannot eat for the rest of the day? To ensure that you haven't gained a quarter of a pound? To see if the binge two days ago was as bad as you thought? To give yourself permission to eat?

Take time to ponder how you use the number on the scale. Is it an excuse to binge or starve? Are you going to judge yourself harshly for what you weigh? Is it going to make or ruin your day? Will it dictate whether or not you spend an extra hour or two in the gym, attend your sister's wedding, purge or take laxatives? Will your scale tell you if you are a good or bad person, as if you're nothing more than poundage?

If your anxiety is sky high unless you weigh yourself, and if this causes you to obsess about what you are or aren't eating, then you might decide that never weighing yourself would result in too much pressure as you journey into uncharted eating territory. Because you don't yet trust yourself or your body when it comes to food, you may feel wildly out of control unless you have an external measure like a scale to rely on. You may need to weigh yourself until you are more comfortable with your new way of eating.

When your eating becomes more "normal," you may no longer feel the need to weigh yourself as often, or at all. If you're used to weighing yourself daily (or more), shoot for once a week, then once a month, then quarterly, and so on until you stop weighing altogether. There may be times when you relapse and binge and temporarily need the security that weighing brings.

Remember, your main focus should be on what you are eating, not on what you weigh. Your goal should be to live comfortably in your body as you let your "normal" eating take care of your weight.

Keep in mind that the scale itself is not your enemy. But neither need it be your lifetime companion. Do "normal" eaters weigh themselves? Some do, and some don't. If they do, you can be sure they're not looking for a magic number to tell them whether it's OK to eat or whether they've been good or bad! A scale is a source of minimal information to them, not a judge and jury. Most important, they weigh themselves only occasionally, not habitually.

The point of avoiding scale-dependence is to help you focus on eating. My hope is that you won't get hung up on the scale issue and make it yet another all-or-nothing dilemma, another right or wrong action, another always-or-never decision. This kind of extreme either-or thinking is exactly what you want to steer clear of—bingeing or dieting, being on or off the wagon, refusing a taste or finishing the whole thing, "I'm good" or "I'm bad." Gently push yourself in the direction of not weighing yourself, but don't make judgments if you do.

On the road to "normal" eating there is no right or wrong to weighing yourself. The only way you'll learn to trust and gain confidence in your decisions is by trial and error. Finding out about weighing yourself is part of this process. Even if you do decide to weigh yourself once in a while, maintain your focus on eating, not what the scale says. Let the rules of "normal" eating guide you to trust your body. If you eat when you're hungry or have a craving, make satisfying food choices, enjoy your food, and stop when you're full or satisfied, you'll be eating exactly what you need. And you will find yourself at a comfortable, healthy weight.

What do you think about exercise?

For disordered eaters, finding a healthy balance of exercise can be a real challenge. Making constructive choices about exercise—neither slacking off nor overdoing it on a regular basis—requires the same tools and processes you're practicing to become a "normal" eater. Building a sound belief system about exercise, listening to and respecting your body, and staying flexible are all keys to a healthy exercise program.

Medical research has repeatedly proven that some form of exercise is necessary to maintain optimum health. Fat, thin, or in-between, you will find that your heart and other body systems work best if you keep them in good condition. So two healthy goals for exercise are to enjoy using and moving your body and to stay fit.

However, if you have an unhealthy relationship with food, you may also have formed an unhealthy relationship with exercise. Perhaps you remember that earlier in this book we talked about having a yes/no disorder, saying yes and no to food and perhaps other life choices inappropriately. Because it's difficult to find a healthy balance, disordered eaters frequently underexercise (too much no) or overexercise (too much yes), which alienates them from their bodies as much as their eating does.

Some factors to consider when you're determining how much or little to exercise include your age, general health, physical condition, medical limitations, lifestyle, and preferences. Forget "No pain, no gain." Whatever exercise you choose, you're more likely to continue it if you enjoy it.

Maintaining a constructive exercise program depends on healthy beliefs about the purpose of physical activity. Rational reasons to exercise include: to lower your cholesterol, tone your muscles, strengthen your bones, stay heart healthy, lose weight sensibly, relax, be fit and well-conditioned, and improve coordination and flexibility. On the other hand, irrational reasons to exercise include: to achieve the "perfect" body, to distract yourself from uncomfortable feelings, to avoid social situations, and to force your body to burn every calorie you consumed all week. To make healthy decisions about the frequency and intensity of exercise, first take a careful look at your purpose and be sure it's consistent with healthy beliefs.

Your beliefs will dictate how you feel about exercise and what you tell yourself about it. Believing that you *need to*, *have to*, *must*, or *should* exercise is not only untrue but counterproductive. Instead of ordering yourself around, try using words such as *want*, *wish*, *desire*, *would like*, or *prefer* and see how much easier it is to reach your exercise goals.

If you're an overexerciser, telling yourself that you *have to* exercise is dangerous because it makes you believe that you have no choice. You may *want* to exercise because you're terrified of gaining weight or feel obsessed to lose more, but you do not *have to* exercise. To break your compulsion and be able to exercise with moderation, you'll need to listen very carefully to your exercise chatter. Then gently guide your thinking around to, *I want to exercise* (a rational statement) in place of the insistent, *I have to exercise* (an irrational statement).

If you're an underexerciser, telling yourself that you *have to* exercise is counterproductive as well because a natural response to that kind of authoritative order is, "I do not, and you can't make me." Words such as *should*, *need to*, *have to*, and *must* all echo the commands we heard in childhood when we had very little choice. You'll be more likely to go for that bike ride or get to the gym or the pool by stating, *I want to exercise*. Using *want* rather than *have to* is a clever trick for decreasing resistance.

Underexercising: What if I can't get myself to exercise?

If you underexercise or don't exercise at all, you probably keep saying you want to begin, while you will find every excuse in the book not to. Or you start, then stop abruptly. Or you gradually start skipping a day here and there, until you haven't been active in weeks or months. Having repeated this start-stop pattern for some time, you end up feeling frustrated, demoralized, undisciplined, and hopeless about ever staying with the program. You procrastinate and call yourself lazy and unmotivated because you're not doing something that's supposedly good for you and that you feel you ought to do.

If this sounds like you, don't despair. You're suffering not from laziness, lack of motivation, or some other serious character defect, but from a severe case of mixed or conflicting feelings. *Whenever your behavior doesn't align with your intent, it means that you're holding two sets of opposing feelings*. What might those feelings be, regarding exercise? Well, on one side of the ledger—the conscious side—you have the benefits, the apparent advantages that result in a sensible desire to exercise: feeling empowered by taking charge of your life, promoting good health, and engaging in behavior that complements your goal of "normal" eating.

The problem is that you're most likely unaware of your feelings on the *other* side of the ledger—the unconscious side. Those contradictory feelings are the reasons you *don't* want to exercise. They lurk just beyond your awareness for a couple of reasons. One is that they make you feel uncomfortable: you don't want to have them because you want to feel positive about exercise. Another is that you're afraid that if you acknowledge them, they'll take over. So you ignore them in the hope they'll go away. But, of course, they never do. They end up pulling the strings from behind the curtain and preventing you from exercising regularly.

Take a minute to think about it. There are valid reasons to avoid exercise: it takes time and planning. Sometimes it costs money. You may be self-conscious about your body or feel clumsy and awkward. You may feel incompetent trying something new and unfamiliar. And any payoff may seem a long way down the road.

Your conflicts can be resolved only when you acknowledge your negative feelings and bring them out into the open. Then your positive feelings won't get split off into your *intent,* or desire to exercise, while your negative feelings get split off into your *behavior,* or desire not to. When you're in touch with both camps, you can make a rational decision that one outweighs the other. At the least, getting in touch with your unconscious feelings will help you get unstuck and decide either to exercise or forgo it until you feel less conflicted.

Overexercising: What if I can't seem to stop?

If you find yourself doing any of the following, consider that you may have an unhealthy relationship with exercise, and you could be overexercising in a way that is be compromising, rather than promoting, good health:

- Running, swimming, walking, or biking many extra miles because you ate more than you thought you should

- Adding weights in excess of your muscle strength solely because you want to burn more calories
- Engaging in aerobic exercise to the point of extreme fatigue, muscle spasm, or lightheadedness
- Continuing to exercise when you're injured or in physical pain
- Never missing a day of exercise no matter what
- Spending more and more time exercising at the expense of other activities
- Forcing yourself to exercise when you're sick and not up to it
- Not permitting yourself to eat when you're hungry or have a craving unless you exercise
- Intensifying your exercise because you put on a pound
- Ignoring relationships because you're spending so much time exercising
- Finding little or no pleasure or a sense of achievement in anything else besides exercise and perfecting your body
- Regularly canceling or avoiding activities you used to enjoy in order to exercise

You may also overexercise to as a way of avoiding uncomfortable feelings. Using exercise for this purpose is similar to the way undereaters focus on calorie counting, eating rituals, and food restriction as distractions from painful or unsettling emotions. What better way to prevent yourself from suffering emotionally than to throw yourself into physical activity, especially when you've convinced yourself that it's good for you! But if you're genuinely in touch with what's going on inside you, you'll notice and respect the difference between pushing yourself to go for a 5-mile hike and having a good old 5-minute cry. There's a huge difference between running off to the gym because you're lonely and can't face the emptiness inside and acknowledging your loneliness, calling a friend, and making plans to get together. I can't say it often enough: There's absolutely no substitute for experiencing painful feelings. They need their own space and time, just as your body needs its own space and time for physical activity.

One last comment for overexercisers. Because popular culture extols exercise, underexercisers often feel heavy censure for their lack of motivation, whereas those addicted to exercise receive considerable reinforcement. This kind of societal validation and encouragement may blind you to your own motives for exercising and make it more difficult to see the damage you're doing to yourself.

As with healthy eating, being true to your feelings and trusting yourself will put you back on the road to healthy exercising. This means using exercise only for constructive reasons, and cuing in to your body's signals for when you've done enough. It also requires sitting with the anxiety that comes from acting in unfamiliar and uncomfortable ways as you cut back your activity to a reasonable, healthy level. When the anxiety arises, simply remind yourself that nothing bad will happen if you exercise less, and that moderating your routine, like "normal" eating, is a healthful way of taking care of yourself.

Applying the rules of "normal" eating, right now!

You've learned a lot by now:

- You know what skills are involved in becoming a "normal" eater.
- You recognize that your beliefs and behavior could use a bit of tinkering.
- You see that feeling your feelings is the only way to stop emotional eating and achieve real happiness.
- You have a sense of what true, effective self-care is.
- You have developed greater awareness of how to deal with challenging food situations.

Most of all, you understand that your body is great and wondrous at any size and that you've been shortchanging it for far too long.

You've got all the pieces of the puzzle in front of you, but maybe you aren't sure if they'll fit together. You're thinking that other people might be able to transform themselves from undereaters or overeaters to "normal" eaters, but that you've got too many hang-ups and other problems, too much baggage, a lousy track record, or not enough motivation. You're scared and excited at the same time.

Whatever you're feeling is OK. Scared and excited is far better than unhappy and hopeless. Of course you don't know everything you need to in order to become a "normal" eater. You'll learn the rest along the way. You don't know everything about life either, but you're not refusing to live because of that! Like all of us, you're feeling your way along and will continue learning until you die. For now, however, you *do* know enough about "normal" eating to move forward. You know your goals and what skills are necessary to reach them. Believe it or not, that's all you need right now.

You've arrived at an incredible choice point in your life, this very instant. You can lay down this book and never look at it again or entertain another thought about "normal" eating. You can grab your highlighter and start rereading this book from page 1. Or you can leave it on your nightstand as a reminder of what's possible. Please don't think that to start down the road to "normal" eating, you have to be ready to transform your whole life all at once. You don't.

The key to change is to start with one action, just one small thing that appeals to you. You could choose from this list or come up with your own ideas.

- Try getting in touch with your physical hunger.
- Call a friend and tell her you have an eating problem.
- Throw out your scale.
- Refuse to compare your body to anyone else's.
- Tell the truth to someone you've been dishonest with.
- Find a therapist and make an appointment.
- Determine whether you have a yes/no or "enough" disorder.
- Get rid of clothes that don't fit and buy some fabulous new outfits.
- Listen hard to your chatter and make sure it's sound and rational.
- Make a list of things you love and hate about your life.
- Have a good cry.
- Look at your body in the mirror and blow yourself a kiss.

- Join a support group to get help with the nondiet approach to eating.
- Face a truth you've been hiding from yourself.
- Trash all your diet books.
- Sit with an upsetting feeling.
- Make an appointment for a physical checkup.
- Have a good laugh over the idea of "good" and "bad" foods.
- Speak up for yourself.

Believe it or not, any one of these actions will move you forward and help you resolve your food and body issues. It doesn't matter where you start; it only matters that you begin *somewhere*. Reading this book is only the beginning.

About the Author

Karen R. Koenig, LICSW, M.Ed. is a psychotherapist, educator, writer, and speaker. A former dieter and compulsive eater, Ms. Koenig has triumphed over her own problems with food. For over 20 years she has taught hundreds of overeaters and undereaters the "normal" eating skills they need to transform their eating and their lives. Along with teaching workshops for the public and for fellow clinicians, she has written essays and articles for *The Boston Globe*, *The Boston Herald*, *Social Work Focus*, and numerous other publications. Visit her website at *www.eatingnormal.com.*

About the Publisher

Since 1980, Gürze Books has specialized in quality information on eating disorders recovery, research, education, advocacy, and prevention. Gürze publishes *Eating Disorders Today*, a newsletter for individuals in recovery and their loved ones, the *Eating Disorders Review,* a clinical newsletter for professionals, and the *Health At Every Size* journal. The company also widely distributes free copies of *The Eating Disorders Resource Catalogue,* which includes listings of books, tapes, and other information. Their website (*www.gurze.com*) is an excellent Internet gateway to treatment facilities, associations, basic facts, and other eating disorder websites.

Order at www.gurze.com
or by phone (760) 434-7533

The Rules of "Normal" Eating is available at bookstores
and libraries and may be ordered directly from the Gürze Books
website, *www.gurze.com*, or by phone (760) 434-7533.

FREE Catalogue

The Eating Disorders Resource Catalogue features books on eating
disorders and related topics, including body image, size acceptance, self-esteem, and more. It includes listings of nonprofit associations and treatment facilities, and it is handed out by thera-
pists, educators, and other health care professionals around the
world.

www.gurze.com

Go to this website for additional resources, including many free
articles, hundreds of eating disorders books, and links to organi-
zations, treatment facilities, and other websites. Gürze Books has
specialized in eating disorders publications and education since
1980.

Eating Disorders Today
A newsletter for individuals in recovery and their loved ones

This compassionate and supportive newsletter combines helpful
facts and self-help advice from respected experts in the field of
eating disorders. Request a sample issue!